Relaxation
for
Children

JENNY RICKARD

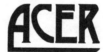

First published 1992
by Collins Dove
Revised and expanded edition published 1994
by The Australian Council for Educational Research Ltd
19 Prospect Hill Road, Camberwell, Melbourne, Victoria 3124, Australia

Line drawings by Marjory Gardner
Cover photograph by Bill Thomas
Cover design by Todd Pierce
Designed by William Hung

Printed by Australian Print Group

The National Library of Australia
Cataloguing-in-Publication data:

Rickard, Jenny.
  Relaxation for children.

  Rev. ed.
  ISBN 0 86431 148 6.

1. Relaxation — Study and teaching (Primary). - 2. Stress in
children — Prevention. 3. Classroom environment. - I. Title.

372.37044

CONTENTS

Foreword

Relaxation for Children is a book that helps fill a heartfelt need of many teachers and parents in our overly stressed society — how best to help our children?

Increasingly, the negative impact of debilitating stress is being recognised as a major drain on health and wellbeing. As a result, more and more adults are turning to relaxation and meditation methods to regain a sense of ease, efficiency and peace in their lives. Having done so, it becomes obvious that to learn these 'anti-stress' skills is like reclaiming our heritage.

For as young children we did have a natural ability to relax, to be joyful, to be positive. In those early years there was a vibrance, joy and optimism that was easy. No effort required here, it was just the way we were.

So what happened? Where did it go? Where did the spontaneous exuberance of youth give way to that tired feeling of always being behind and having to be playing 'catch-up'.

It would seem that in the business of life, faced with limited means of coping with life's difficulties and traumas, we lost our natural ease. In its place came feelings of stress, of not being good enough, of losing our way.

It is an unhappily common adult experience to relate to all this, to realize that we become caught up in self-defeating habits in seeking what is missing in drugs or other empty diversions.

So it is delightful to observe, in fact, to be part of helping adults to regain that natural, joyous ease. To find what they are really looking for.

For this is the good news — peace of mind can be found. It can be learnt and sustained in a personally satisfying way. In fact, for many adults, this learning becomes a life-changing, sometimes even life-saving path to follow.

But then, what of our children? For them, there is an even better hope, the prospect that they may never even lose it.

However, it does seem clear — the evidence of the past proves it to us — that if there is no active intervention, many children will develop stress responses that become unhealthy and unhappy. Left unchecked, this is likely to diminish both home and school life.

Grace and I have four children, currently 10-15 years old. Our own observation is that a great deal of class time is often taken up dealing with the impact of negative stress. Frequently it seems that the attempts to control the associated disruptions and inefficiencies actually result in reinforcing the negative patterns.

This is where relaxation and meditation techniques offer fresh possibilities. The stress cycle can be broken directly and children can learn a new, personal lifeskill of relaxation, ease and inner peace.

This is where Jenny Rickard's *Relaxation for Children* is a godsend. First, it clearly details how children can learn to relax and harmonize their bodies. In so doing, they can maintain their natural relaxed state. This physically-based lifeskill has the added bonus of heightening physical achievement, as a stress free body is clear to perform at its best — a boon for all sporting activity.

Secondly, the book can help children to learn about maintaining their own space. What this means, in its true essence, is to know yourself — deeply. For we adults this may sound rather grand and complex. For children it is a simple inner experience — a direct experience of who they really are.

With a direct experience of this inner self, comes a quiet confidence, an assurance, a warm inner glow. A feeling of belonging, of having purpose and meaning. This translates for children into a clear view of their own boundaries, of what is true, fair and reasonable, of what is important in life.

Those who are smart enough to read and apply the principles of this book will learn a lifeskill or teach it to their children and this will provide the basis for a good life. Naturally this does not mean that such a life will be free of ups and downs, good times and bad. But it does mean that there will be available a readily accessible, personally satisfying means of firstly coping with life, but then — more importantly — being able to live it to the full.

I have given a copy of this book to each of my children. I recommend it to all teachers and parents.

Ian Gawler
March 1994
Author of *You Can Conquer Cancer* and *Peace of Mind*

ACKNOWLEDGEMENTS

The inspiration for developing this program came from the 1984 Grade Six students of St Francis Xavier Primary School, Box Hill, and in particular, Michael Vozzo.

The motivational force for the actual writing was Carol Blackett-Smith, my colleague, dear friend, and critic.

Encouragement came from many, many people, in particular, my husband, Raymond, my daughters, Danielle and Ellise, my mother, and my husband's parents.

Practical assistance came from the many students who have participated in the program, their parents and teachers and other professionals who have read and used the program.

PREFACE

'Hey, Mrs Rickard!' I looked towards the gate where Michael, a not-so-willing Grade Six boy, was lining up for his bus. 'Mrs Rickard, do you know what? That relaxation stuff you gave us was great. I had to do my entrance exam on Saturday and I remembered the breathing and some other stuff and . . . it worked.' This comment made my day. It reinforced my belief in the value of teaching students how to relax.

My initial interest in relaxation began many years ago, when I was preparing for the birth of my first child. I adapted and used the skills I learnt at pre-natal classes in other situations. Later I learnt a wider range of skills, first as a student of psychology and then as a student of yoga. Gradually I added my own ideas and practices.

My interest in teaching relaxation techniques to children was aroused through my work as an educationist. I had received many requests from teachers to work with them on social skills and self-esteem programs for students. For many groups, it became apparent that a relaxation activity would be appropriate, and so I decided, somewhat hesitantly, to devote a segment of each session to having what I then called a 'Quiet Time'.

From these experiences I began to develop and refine a framework for teaching children to relax. This framework is built on two essential concepts: (1) body harmony, which is achieved when the inside and the outside parts of the body work together to achieve relaxation, and (2) creating one's own physical, seeing, hearing and mind space. It is these two concepts, with their associated skills, that I believe have made the program successful and distinguish it from other approaches.

The material presented in this text has been used and developed with many groups of students over the past eight years. This new edition includes ideas and suggestions given to me from people all over Australia who have attended my workshops and used the first edition of the book. To these people I give a big thank you for your enthusiasm and encouragement, and for understanding the importance of empowering children.

Jenny Rickard
1994

Part One

INTRODUCTION

My prime motivation for writing this text is my belief that relaxation skills should be viewed as a valuable 'life skill', like many others that we learn in childhood, such as learning how to ride a bike or swim. These are useful and enjoyable activities and ones which stay with us for life and can, in fact, be life-savers if they are learnt well. So too with relaxation skills. If we learn them early in life and learn them well, they can become building blocks on which we can develop further skills at a later stage. They can also provide us with positive automatic responses in many frightening or overwhelming situations. They can empower us and positively affect the way we respond to important events in our life.

In considering other reasons for teaching children relaxation skills, there needs to be some understanding of the role of stress and how it affects children.

In a clinical sense, *stress* refers to the state of arousal we feel as we go about our daily life. Stress is the motivation we need to get us going; it is an energy force we can use effectively. However, if we have too many things to do, if they are beyond our experience, or too hard or too new to us, then the arousal we feel is likely to make us uncomfortable. We can begin to experience the negative side of stress. We become *distressed.*

Stress is best understood as an interaction between the demands of the environment and the individual's coping skills (Charles Spielberger 1979). *Distress* is the gap between those demands and the individual's coping skills.

The second point to understand about stress is that it is a *process.* It does not operate in isolation. Past experience and actions, thoughts, feelings, self-esteem and physical health are all components of the stress process.

If we acknowledge these two points, we can begin to understand how learning relaxation skills can be an important way of increasing children's coping skills. These skills will help increase their self-esteem and the likelihood that they will respond positively to the challenges they are required to meet.

For example, a new task could be having to read at a school assembly. The child will start thinking and feeling processes which, in turn, will govern the action outcomes. If these thinking and feeling processes are negative and create strong physical reactions, then the child needs to acknowledge them and have some way of dealing with them, such as using positive self-talk or relaxation skills. These in turn will help the child carry out the required task in a positive and confident manner. Thus self-esteem, and the likelihood that she or he may approach other new tasks positively, have been increased. Like the Grade Six boy, Michael, the child becomes less anxious and feels empowered to perform the required task.

Another reason for teaching children relaxation skills is to help them cope with strong emotional responses. Children, like adults, will hold groups of muscles tight when experiencing such emotions as fear, anger, anxiety, excitement or worry. It is useful for them to be able to learn to locate these feelings in their bodies, to talk to that part and to let the muscle tension go. It is very difficult to stay angry if we have relaxed face, neck, shoulder and back muscles.

The program is especially useful in that it enables children to respond to a very common directive given to them by many adults: 'Relax, take it easy, don't get uptight'. Teaching children relaxation skills empowers them: they know what they can do.

It is important to appreciate that relaxation is also a *process*. This needs to be recognized and reflected in teaching relaxation skills. There is a preparation stage followed by a routine in which the last stage is Quiet Time. This is where one lies or sits quietly and listens to an imagery tape or quiet music. To get the most benefit from this process, children and adults alike must have some knowledge of their own bodies and develop a number of specific skills that will help them to achieve a calm, peaceful and relaxed state. An approach to developing this understanding and these skills forms the content of the program presented in this book.

The material is structured in such a way that it removes any 'mystique' and makes relaxation skills available to all interested people. It draws on the three domains through which we experience life: the cognitive, the affective and the physical (that is: thinking, feeling and doing) and combines them in the learning of new tasks.

Whether you are a general reader, a teacher, health practitioner or interested parent, I know you will find this book a valuable resource, and one that will provide you with a practical, easy and enjoyable approach to teaching children relaxation skills.

Aims of the Program

The aims of this relaxation program are:
- to increase students' coping skills so that they can respond positively to the demands of their environment;
- to build students' awareness and understanding of our wonderful bodies and how they work;

• to teach students how to make the whole body calm and peaceful.

The skills taught are based on the two concepts of *body harmony* and *one's own space*. As the students develop these skills they begin to master the technique of 'getting the whole body to be calm and peaceful'. The concepts and the skills taught are described below.

Body Harmony

Body harmony is when the inside and outside parts of the body work together towards one goal: relaxation. To achieve body harmony, the students need:

• to be able to identify and locate the main body parts. They need to be able to recognize how these body parts feel and what they look like — for example, my fingers are short, they feel soft, bony, and so on;
• to identify major muscle groups, know how muscles work and how muscles feel when they are tense or relaxed;
• to understand how they breathe and learn to use different breathing techniques which will help them relax and revitalize their bodies.

One's Own Space

The concept of one's own space has two functions. First, it acts as a poetic symbol, helping students to concentrate and shut off the distractions of the busy world around them. This is the first step to relaxing. One's own space is where one cannot be disturbed, where one shuts out the sights and sounds of the people and things around one, and ceases to think of everyday matters. The children are taught the skill of consciously withdrawing from their surroundings for a short time.

The students learn:

• how to create and use their own physical, seeing, hearing and mind space;
• to create positive, calming and peaceful images and use them in a variety of ways to 'make their bodies calm and peaceful'.

The second function of this concept is that it acts as a group rule, so that it becomes unacceptable to disturb others by 'going into another person's space'; in other words, by talking, nudging them or distracting them in any other way.

Format of the Sessions

This is a structured program, consisting of ten sessions, each of which builds on the work from the preceding session. This work is reviewed and briefly discussed before commencing the next session.

Each session has six sequential stages in which students work at their own pace so that they will become familiar with and confident in understanding and using their new skills.

1.   Joining Together

When joining together a 'working circle' is made; this is a way of showing that the group will join together and cooperate in helping each other to learn the relaxation skills and practise them. It is a time to quieten down and clear the mind.

2.   Review Time

At the beginning of each session, the leader and students discuss how they have practised the skills they learnt in the previous session. Time can also be spent discussing the key concepts and revising skills.

3.   Instruction Time

In this stage the students are introduced to the main concepts of the program and the skills they need to acquire to be able to make their bodies and minds calm and peaceful.

4.   Practical Activities

Here the students practise skills. They stretch and loosen their muscles, make their bodies tight and floppy, deepen and slow their breathing, experiment with getting into their own space, and use imagery to help them in all the activities.

Note: In most sessions, stages 3 and 4 are combined.

5.   Quiet Time

Quiet time is when the students get into their 'own space' and use imagery to help them to become calm and peaceful and to feel great about themselves.

6.   Reflection Time

This is the final stage of the session when the students discuss how they felt doing the activities, and they are given positive feedback about their progress. The students also comment on how they will practise and when they will use the skills before the next session.

Note: Practice points for students are suggested in each session. These can be done between sessions, both in class time and at home. Young children especially gain a lot from sharing their relaxation skills with their family. Alternatively, these suggestions can serve as ideas for 'refresher' activities in the classroom.

Role of the Teacher

The teacher's role becomes that of a leader who is also a participant with the children in the group. The teacher models appropriate behaviour for the group, talking about her or his responses to the exercises and sharing her or his feelings with the group. In fact, the success of the relaxation program depends very much on the willingness of the teacher to participate in this way, for she or he thus encourages the children to take the risk of talking about their feelings. Encouragement, acceptance and use of positive reinforcement after each exercise or activity are implicit.

The teacher needs to try out all the exercises and be able to demonstrate them to the group, not just talk about them.

The teacher sets the tone for the sessions by being accepting of each child's response to the material. Individual difficulties should be dealt with quietly and with the least distraction for the rest of the group.

Where two teachers are able to participate in the group, both benefit: the leader gets direct feedback, while the associate experiences the program at first hand and has the opportunity to learn from her or his peer.

Procedures

This section sets out those procedures that should be followed in the program and some practical hints to ensure the smooth running of sessions.

The Room

The room should be large enough for all students to lie on the floor without touching each other — with about a one-metre space between them. The room needs to be carpeted, warm, private, away from noise and with a door that closes! Put up a sign: 'Do not disturb — relaxation in progress'. There should be as few visual distractions in the room as possible, and drapes or blinds should be drawn.

Equipment

- A good-quality cassette recorder or CD player.
- A selection of taped music suitable for a calm and relaxing atmosphere. Some suggestions for suitable music are provided in Part Five.
- An overhead projector.
- A power point, and double adaptor if necessary.
- Charts of the overheads for use as aids to the teacher (optional).

Clothing

It is important that the children be warm and comfortable. No special apparel is needed, although children should be encouraged to wear loose clothing. Shoes are removed before each session. Children may like to bring a blanket.

Most importantly, if children suffer from asthma or allergies, they need a pillowcase, towel or small rug to put under their face when they lie on the floor.

Teacher's Voice

The teacher's tone of voice is very important. It needs to be calm and reassuring. It should be firm, but not too loud. Be aware of your natural voice pitch and try to keep your voice low and even. Speak with expression to emphasize words when appropriate. Repeat key words or phrases two or three times. It helps if you articulate clearly and try to slow down your rate of speech. It may sound unnatural to you, but to your audience, it will be just right. Remember: slow ... steady ... clear.

Routine

The key to successful relaxation sessions with children of all ages is routine. When a routine is followed and used with the two rules (see Rules on page 9), discipline issues do not arise. Establish a clear routine with the students so that they always know what they have to do, both on entering and leaving the room. In addition, make sure that the students are in a comfortable position and are able to pay attention to you before introducing a new activity.

(a) Entering the Room

Students remove shoes before entering the room and quietly sit in their own space. It is helpful to have quiet music playing in the background. Have one or two pieces of music that the students will identify as 'quiet music'. When all the students are in the room, begin the session by asking them to form a circle quietly and join hands.

(b) The Working Circle

Forming the circle signals the commencement of the session and symbolizes the commitment of each person to the group. It is also a time for the students and leader(s) to quieten down and clear their minds of the day's activities. Use a simple imagery exercise that helps to clear the mind. For example, direct students to close their eyes and think about the things they have been doing during the day. Then, ask them to put these things into a big paper bag, to tie it up tight and take it and put it outside the door. This exercise can be introduced in the second or third session.

When working with a large group of students, it is more effective to have an inner and outer circle. The group leaders sit interspersed among the children.

(c)   Finishing Routine
The finishing routine brings the students out of the relaxed state of the 'quiet time'. Finishing routines are spelt out in the sessions.

(d)   Closure
This is a formal way of ending the sessions. Closure is most important as it sets a relaxed mood that will stay with the students when they leave the session.

A format for the closure is given in Sessions One and Two. This can be used for concluding all ten sessions, thus ensuring that the students leave the room in a quiet and calm way.

Rules
The program has two very simple rules. It is important to spend time talking about these rules and clearly state them in the first two or three sessions.

Rule 1:   During a relaxation session, students must stay in their own physical, hearing and seeing space. If students are having difficulty in attending to the session, or are disruptive, remind them that they are getting into someone else's space (physical, hearing, seeing). This concept is fully discussed in Session One.

Rule 2:   If students are having difficulty or feel uncomfortable with any part of the session, then they may choose just to sit quietly and calmly in their space until they feel able to join in again.

When Students Experience Difficulty
Some students initially may have difficulty with:
1 closing their eyes; or
2 choosing a comfortable sitting or lying position.

Closing Eyes
For many people, the idea of closing their eyes in a public situation is very risky and may pose a threat. If a child in your group is having this difficulty, gently and quietly encourage her or him to try shutting the eyes a little at a time, gradually lengthening the time the eyes are closed. Encourage the child just to listen to your voice or the music, and not to focus on the fact that the eyes are closed.

Another difficulty that can be encountered is closing eyes too tightly, so that they are screwed up and therefore tense. This will sometimes happen if a student is trying too hard or is very tense or apprehensive.

The best way to deal with this is first to use the words 'gently/slowly, close your eyes'. Second, touch the student quietly on the forehead and say 'relax your eyes, have them gently closed'. Doing this a couple of times should be enough to help the student.

Choosing a Comfortable Position

You might need to give some students individual help to find a comfortable position. If they have a tendency to move parts of the body or just become restless, quietly and gently touch them and stay near them until they can relax a little more. You might like to suggest that they sit up in a comfortable position and just listen. This same procedure would also apply to students who get a fit of coughing or the hiccups.

Avoid at all cost, drawing attention to a student who is having some difficulty; deal with it on an individual level, using a quiet approach.

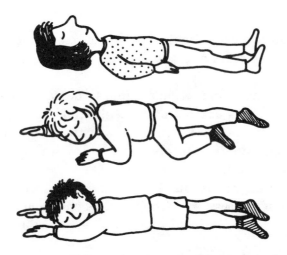

Comfortable Positions for Relaxation

Session Length and Timing of Exercises

Although it is difficult to be precise, most sessions will usually take about forty-five minutes to an hour. Times for exercises, pauses and so on, are suggested, but you might like to vary them for your particular group. Do make notes of your variations, as you can then be consistent. It is also very helpful if you rehearse and time the exercises yourself, to get an idea of how the activity feels and what is involved.

Participation

Like any other lesson or program, success depends on how much those involved are prepared to put into it. As leader and participant, the teacher has to take responsibility for enabling the whole class to participate by providing a good model for the group. Experience has shown that the most successful sessions are those where the group leaders and the students have been co-workers and have shared their experiences. Leaders need to be willing to share their feelings and thoughts so that the group will in turn be prepared to contribute.

Preparation

Sessions go smoothly when the group leader is prepared. The room, the charts, overheads, tapes, overhead projector and cassette recorder all need to be ready before the start of the session. A missing extension cord can ruin a session, and no one is relaxed if you have to go chasing one! Equally, it is very important that session notes have been read carefully and, if necessary, cue cards have been made. Being well prepared and familiar with the material will ensure that the session flows with relaxed ease. Of course, as routines are established, things will run smoothly.

Creativity

When using this material in schools, teachers have found that it is readily extended to other areas of their curriculum. For example, the skills of body harmony can be developed in drama, health education and science. A creative teacher will find limitless ways of introducing and extending this material.

Music

The 'quiet time' activities in Sessions One to Six all require music. The music needs to be quiet and restful, with little variation in tempo. Music for the 'quiet time' and other parts of the program is suggested in Part Five.

Guided Imagery

Guided imagery is introduced in Session Seven and practised in subsequent sessions. A spoken dialogue has been provided for each session, but if you don't feel confident in using it, the names of some good commercial tapes are provided in Part Five.

Listen to the tapes before you use them to ensure that they will suit your group.

You might like to make your own tapes, drawing on the suggestions in Sessions Eight, Nine and Ten and Part Three.

Use of This Book

The Sessions

The ten sessions in the book follow the six-stage sequence described on page 6. An outline of the material in each session is provided in the Program Summary.

At the beginning of each session are listed:

- the aims of the session;
- teaching aids required;
- vocabulary used in the session;
- knowledge and techniques taught in the session.

Overheads used in the session are provided as blackline masters at the end of the book.

A **verbatim script** is provided for many of the exercises. You might like to follow these until you feel confident with the material. They are a basis only, to be modified to suit your purposes and your own creativity.

Discussion Points and **Practice Points** are listed under stage 6: Reflection Time. These are suggestions only. You will find in practice that discussion and suggestions for practice activities will arise naturally out of each session. The same applies to the **Classroom Activities** listed at the end of each session.

Other Materials

A **workbook** for students is provided on blackline masters at the end of the book (see Part Five). This should be worked through at home so that the students have the opportunity to share their knowledge and skills with their family. It can be introduced when it feels appropriate.

If you are running a program, it is strongly suggested that you hold a 'Parent Evening' so that you maximize the opportunity for parent support and participation. Part Five provides notes for parents, a structure for a parent information workshop and suggestions for overheads. The student workbook can be introduced on this evening so that parents can work through it with their children.

Part Three contains activities for short routines, stretching, loosening up, breathing and guided imagery exercises.

Part Four contains ideas for parents and activities for home.

Part Five contains an outline for teachers running a parent workshop, music, tapes with spoken dialogue for imagery exercises, list of books for further reading, a certificate and handout notes for parents after children have completed the course.

Part Two

PROGRAM SUMMARY

Session One

1. **Outline of Program Routines**
2. **The Working Circle**
3. **Introduction**
   Name Game
4. **Instruction and Practice Time**
   The Concept of Body Harmony
   Activity: Body Awareness
   The Concept of One's Own Space
   Activity: Getting into One's Own Space
5. **Quiet Time**
   Learning to Close the Eyes
   The Finishing Routine
6. **Reflection Time**

Session Two

1. **Joining Together**
2. **Review Time**
   The Concept of One's Own Space
   The Concept of Body Harmony
3. & 4. **Instruction and Practice Time**
   Body Awareness Activity
   Body Quiz
5. **Quiet Time**
   Getting into Your Own Space
6. **Reflection Time**

Session Three

1. **Joining Together**
2. **Review Time**
   Body Awareness
3. & 4. **Instruction and Practice Time**
   Introduction to Muscle Awareness
   Muscle Exercises
5. **Quiet Time**
   Making the Whole Body Floppy
6. **Reflection Time**

Session Four

1. **Joining Together**

2.   **Review Time**
Muscles

3. & 4. **Instruction and Practice Time**
Introduction to 'Ouch' Spots
Activity: Systematic Relaxation of Muscles
Loosening Up Muscles

5.   **Quiet Time**
Relaxing Muscles

6.   **Reflection Time**

Session Five

1.   **Joining Together**

2.   **Review Time**
Concepts of Body Harmony and One's Own Space
Muscle Work and Checking for 'Ouch' Spots

3. & 4. **Instruction and Practice Time**
Introduction to Stretching Techniques
Awareness of Breathing
Relax, Slow, and Deep Breathing Exercises

5.   **Quiet Time**
Slow, Deep Breathing

6.   **Reflection Time**

Session Six

1.   **Joining Together**

2.   **Review Time**
Awareness of Breathing
Relax and Slow Breathing

3. & 4. **Instruction and Practice Time**
Climbing Stretch Activity
Cleansing and Energy Breathing Exercises

5.   **Quiet Time**
Energy Breathing

6.   **Reflection Time**

Session Seven

1.   **Joining Together**

2.   **Review Time**
Review of Knowledge and Skills that Help Us Relax

3. & 4. **Instruction and Practice Time**
Brick Wall Stretch
Cleansing Breathing
Introduction to the Concept of Imagery

5.   **Quiet Time**
Creating an Image of One's Own Special Space

6.   **Reflection Time**

Session Eight

1.   **Joining Together**
2.   **Review Time**
      Key Components of Relaxation
      Imagery Exercise
3. & 4. **Instruction and Practice Time**
      Stretching Exercises
      Breathing Exercises
5.   **Quiet Time**
      Development of Image of One's Special Space
6.   **Reflection Time**

Session Nine

1.   **Joining Together**
2.   **Review Time**
      Key Components of Relaxation
3. & 4. **Instruction and Practice Time**
      Loosening Up Activities
      Cleansing Breathing
      Scalp Massage
      Muscle Exercise
5.   **Quiet Time**
      Guided Imagery — 'Floating on a Cloud'
6.   **Reflection Time**

Session Ten

1.   **Joining Together**
2.   **Review Time**
      Practice Activities
3. & 4. **Instruction and Practice Time**
      Scalp Massage
      Muscle Exercise: Body Scan for 'Ouch' Spots
      Breathing Exercise
5.   **Quiet Time**
      Guided Imagery — 'A Visit to a Magic Island'
6.   **Reflection Time**
7.   **Presentation of Certificates**

SESSION ONE

Aims
- to introduce the routines;
- to give an overview of the sessions and then to introduce the two major concepts — body harmony and one's own space;
- to get to know each other.

Teaching Aids
cassette recorder, music tape, overhead projector, Overheads 1–6, small reusable name tags for each student, larger name tags with names clearly printed in large letters.

Vocabulary
relax, relaxation, distract, interrupt, physical, concept, harmony, peaceful, gently.

Knowledge/Techniques
concept of body harmony, body parts, concept of one's own space, entering and finishing routines.

1. Outline of Program Routines
Before beginning this session, explain to the students that you want them to enter and leave the room quietly. They are to remove their shoes, enter quietly and sit on the floor in a circle, listening to the quiet music until everyone has joined the circle. Practise this. Then introduce the Working Circle.

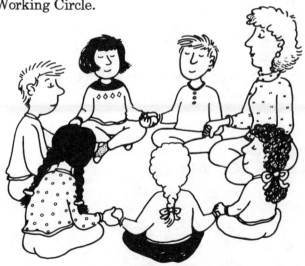

The Working Circle

2. The Working Circle

At the beginning of each session, the students gently join hands to make links in their circle. (See the illustration opposite.) This shows that they all join and work together. It also helps them to slow down and be still before beginning their work. Practise this once with them.

3. Introduction

Discuss with the students the purpose of the sessions: to learn new skills and to learn how to relax. Introduce the definition of relaxation. Show Overhead 1.

OH 1

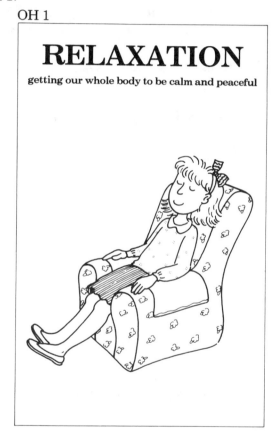

RELAXATION

getting our whole body to be calm and peaceful

Give students a brief overview of each session. Explain the purpose of each stage of the session: review time, learning and practice of skills, quiet time and so on.

It is a very good idea if you are working with a group of students who do not know you or each other to begin this first session with a 'Getting to know you activity' such as the one below.

Name game

1. Ask students to sit in a large circle. Read out each name from the large name cards and give the cards to the students.

2. Ask students to draw around their names some things they enjoy or things that are special to them. (Allow only a few minutes.)

3. Ask students to share what they have drawn on the card with another person.

4. Ask the students to introduce their partner to the group and to tell the group one thing they have learned about that person, for example, 'This is Anne and she likes cats'. The name cards are then placed in front of each person.

5. Place the small, reusable name tags face down in the centre of the circle. Select a child to choose a card. She or he then reads out the name on the card and presents it to that person, who in turn takes a card. When all are read, the cards are then pinned on to the children.

N.B. It is useful to use these name tags for the first few weeks until everyone gets to know each other.

4. Instruction and Practice Time

Body Harmony

Introduce the concept of body harmony — where all the parts of our body work together. Show Overhead 2.

OH 2

BODY HARMONY

- knowing the parts of your body and how they can work together;

- getting the inside and outside body parts working together so you can be **calm** and **peaceful.**

Group discussion: What do we mean by our body? What do bodies do? What are some parts of our bodies? How should we care for our bodies? For example, treat them gently and with care.

OH 3

OH 4

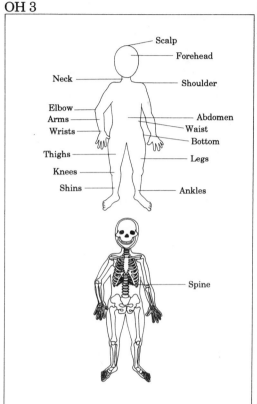
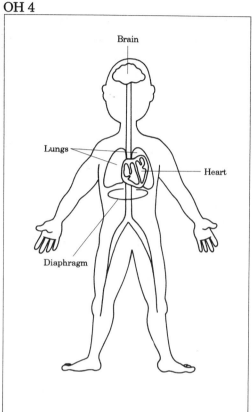

Summarize the discussion and extend it to a discussion of outside and inside parts, using Overhead 3 to show the outside parts, (that is, those we can see, like arms, legs, head and so on), and Overhead 4 to show the inside parts, (those that cannot be seen, such as heart, lungs, brain, muscles, joints, spine).

The rationale for teaching about the parts of the body is that the whole body is involved in relaxation. This is particularly important with the inside parts: the muscles, the heart, the lungs and especially, the brain.

Tell students:

When we learn to relax we are actually learning how to get the parts we can see and the parts that we cannot see to work together so that we become calm and peaceful. This is what we call body harmony.

Show Overhead 2 again.

Activity: Body Awareness

The first activity is designed to discover how well the students know their bodies and to increase their awareness of their body parts. Tell students:

Stand, with your feet apart. Press your feet firmly into the carpet, first one then the other. Wiggle your toes, then press them into the carpet, one after the other. Touch the back of your legs. Feel them gently. Now, point to your knees, your thighs, your hips, your waist, your chest.

Find your heart. Feel it beating. Point to where your lungs are … move your shoulders up and down …

Think about your spine … where is it? See it in your mind's eye … now gently, point to the top of your spine … now the bottom of your spine.

Think about the joints of your body … now touch one … wrist, elbow, knee, or ankle.

Concentrate on your face. Can you try to raise your eyebrows? Wrinkle your nose? Clench your teeth? Where is your tongue now? Can you move it over your teeth?

Move your head slowly to one side and then the other. Put your chin on your chest, then slowly point it up into the air. Now chin down and look to the front.

Well done! Now you are a little more aware of the inside and outside parts of the body.

Review why being aware of these parts is important for learning body harmony: to know our body parts so that we can get them to work together. With the students sitting comfortably, introduce the second concept, one's own space.

One's Own Space

Introduce this concept by first discussing with the group the ways in which they already have their own space for when they need to be by themselves, for example, their bedroom, cubby, favourite chair. Encourage them to think of other places, spaces, which are special for them.

Introduce to the group the idea that they can also create this kind of space to help them to relax. This is what is referred to as one's own space. Show Overheads 5 and 6.

OH 5

OH 6

GETTING INTO MY OWN SPACE

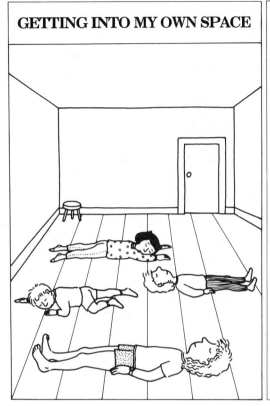

MY OWN SPACE

· creating my *own*
   – physical
   – seeing
   – hearing
   – mind
   space;

· being able to stay in my own space so that I can be **calm** and **peaceful**.

While showing Overhead 6 comment on the four aspects of this concept.

We need to have our own physical space, where we cannot touch anyone else, or be touched.

We need to have our own hearing space, where we cannot hear others or make noises that will go into someone else's space.

We need to have our own seeing space, where we are not distracted or do things that will distract others. The best way to create our own seeing space is to close our eyes gently.

We need to have our own mind space, where we are no longer thinking of everyday things. Our mind is blank, like a clean sheet of paper.

Activity: Getting into One's Own Space

The children spread out quietly and find their own space. They may either sit or lie there. Make sure that they are comfortable. If they are leaning against anything, they may become stiff. If they lie, they need to be flat on their back, on their tummy or on one side. Take the time to check each student.

Check the *physical space*. Are they touching anyone? Are they comfortable? Let them think about getting into their own space. Ask them if they feel tight or stiff. If so, ask them to try to let go of the tightness.

Check the *seeing space*. Are any students looking around? Watching you? If so, you are in their seeing space. Ask them to close their eyes. This is the best way to block out all visual stimuli, and not run the risk of distracting or being distracted by another person. If students are not ready to close the eyes completely, let them half close them and look down.

Finally, check *hearing space*. Is there noise from others, either inside or outside the room? If so, ask students to push it to the back of their minds, and just to listen to your voice and the music. Remind them not to distract others by making any noise themselves.

Finally, check the *mind space*. Have they cleared their minds? Are they clear, like a blank sheet?

In a calm voice, say:

You are now in your own space. Just stay there for a few seconds. (Allow about one minute.) *I am going to ask you to close your eyes. Very slowly and gently, shut your eyes and listen to me counting. When I get to 10, slowly and gently open your eyes.* (Count slowly to 10.) *Well done! Shut your eyes again, slowly. I am going to count to 20, and when I get there, slowly and gently open your eyes. 1...2...3* (etc.) *Well done.*

5. Quiet time

Learning to close the eyes

Direct students to remain in their own space and introduce the activity of Quiet Time by telling students that this is the time in the session when they will practise getting into their own space and use imagery to assist them to become calm and peaceful. Say:

This time, we are going to close our eyes and listen to some music.

Slowly and gently, close your eyes and just quietly and calmly listen to the music.

Leave the music on for about two minutes and take note of any students who may be having difficulty and give them assistance. (See Introduction, p. 9.)

The Finishing Routine

Soon we are going to end this session. It will be done to a count of 10. When I start to count, I want you to bring your thoughts back to this room. Feel yourself lying or sitting on the floor and listen to my voice. Move your fingers and toes gently, and slowly open your eyes. 1...2...3...4...5. Just lie still with your eyes open. Now I will finish counting to 10. By the time I reach 10, all of you who have been lying will be sitting up. Slowly and gently, start to sit up. 6...7...8...9...10. Now slowly stand up and gently give your bodies a stretch. On tip toes, reach up to the ceiling and stretch ... stretch. Now, come slowly back down and just stand quietly. Well done!

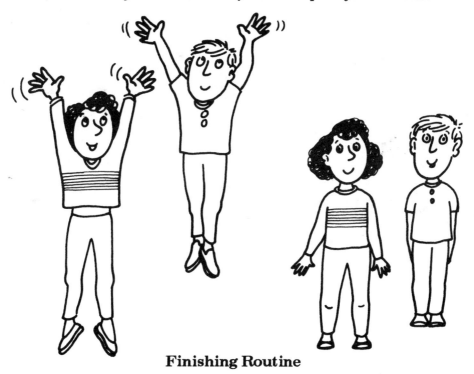

Finishing Routine

6. Reflection Time

Discussion Points

Bring the students back into the Working Circle and discuss the following points:

- **Definition of Relaxation:** What is it?
- Ask how the exercises felt. Did people feel calm and peaceful? Give assurance to others that it takes time and practice to relax, and that with each session, they will all be better able to get their bodies to be calm and peaceful.
- **Concept of Body Harmony:** review meaning.
- **Concept of One's Own Space:** review meaning.
- Seek comment from the students.

Practice Points

Encourage the children to practise their own 'quiet times'.

Closure

This is the last part of each session. The students remain in their working circle. Play some soft music, and ask the students to sit quietly, with their eyes closed, and to think over what they have done in the session. After about 60 seconds, tell them that it is time to finish and leave the group. The students open their eyes, stand up slowly, and quietly leave the room.

Classroom Activities

- Working individually, students fill in the names of parts of the body on a blank outline of the human body.
- In small groups, students trace and cut out a full-size figure. They label the parts, or the teacher provides a set of cards with the names of body parts on them, and the children play a game of pinning on the cards.
- As a class have a Body Quiz. For example, point to your heart, head, etc. or play 'Simon Says', according to the age/temperament of your class.
- A writing or discussion activity. Children describe their own parts of the body. For example, 'My hand has ... it feels like ...'.
- Body Measuring. An activity for pairs, small groups or homework with family, and later discussion in class.
- **Quiet Times:** As teacher, organize a set, formal time each day when the students sit or lie in a comfortable position for a few minutes. Ideally, this should be at the same time each day, to become part of the class routine. During this quiet time, the children practise closing their eyes and shutting out any noise. Encourage the children to give themselves their own quiet time.
- **Body Knowledge:** Set body quizzes for homework, suggesting that students do these in bed, first thing in the morning or last thing at night.

SESSION TWO

Aims
- to revise the two key concepts — body harmony and one's own space;
- to develop the concept of body harmony, by creating awareness of the parts of one's body.

Teaching Aids
overhead projector, Overheads 3–6, music tape for 'Quiet Time', cassette recorder.

Vocabulary
relax, relaxation, distract, interrupt, physical, concept, harmony, peaceful, gently.

Knowledge/Techniques
awareness of body parts, getting into one's own space.

1. Joining Together
Form the Working Circle allowing time for the students to quieten down and clear their minds of the day's activities.

2. Review Time

The Concept of One's Own Space
Discuss with the group what this means, and its purpose (a space we create in which we can be by ourselves). Show Overheads 5 and 6.

Ask the students what is meant by our own *physical space*, our own *hearing space*, our own *seeing space* and our own *mind space*.

Practise quickly sitting in one's own space.

The Concept of Body Harmony
Discuss with the students what this means, and what happens when our bodies are in harmony? How should we treat our bodies? What do we need to know about our bodies to achieve body harmony? Show Overheads 3 and 4.

Sum up this review time with:

When we relax we get those body parts we can see and those we cannot see to work together, so that we become calm and peaceful.

Today, we are going to do another activity which will help each of us to get to know our bodies better. There is one very important thing we need to remember and that is: our bodies are wonderful and so we must learn to treat them gently.

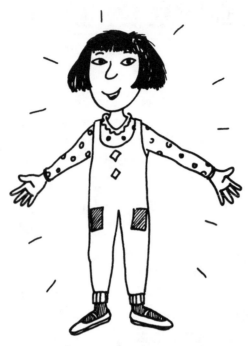

3. & 4. Instruction and Practice Time

Body Awareness Activity

Note: The format of this session will vary according to the age of the group of students. Older children can be directed to find their own space and to sit or lie in it. They are then directed to use their minds to help picture the parts of their body. Encourage them also to take their minds into a particular part of their body and to really visualize it and feel it in their minds.

Younger children can find their own space and stand in it. Get them to show you various body parts by some appropriate actions. Say:

Where is your head? Point to it … Give it a gentle shake and a gentle nod. Take your hand and gently feel its shape. Is it hard? Soft? Put your hand at the back of your head and now put it on the front of your head. Point to where your brain is.

Where is your neck? Point to it and put your hands gently around it. Feel its shape. Hold your neck while moving your head from side to side slowly … Now up and down slowly.

Where is your forehead? Touch it. Now touch your cheeks, your ears, eyes, nose, mouth, and chin.

Let's find your shoulders … move them up and down slowly … become aware of each shoulder.

Now point to your chest, your abdomen. It's just below your chest. Now point to your tummy. Gently pat your chest, your abdomen and your tummy.

Allow time now for the students to reflect on what they have been doing. Ask them to share their thoughts. Have they learnt or felt anything different? It is important for them to share their feelings. Ask them what they have learnt by doing the actions. Then resume.

Raise your arms, up, up. Let them down gently. Hold up your hands ... move your fingers ... make them dance gently ... feel your fingers ... now lower your hands.

Touch one elbow. Now the other one. Make a circle of your fingers around your wrists ... Hold for 1...2... Move your wrist up and down ... feel around your wrist.

As best you can, point to your back ... Now put your hands on your bottom. Can you touch your spine?

Now for your legs. Touch your thighs and hold for two seconds ... 1...2... now your knees ... 1...2... now your shins. They are just below your knees. 1...2... Shake one foot, now the other. Point to your ankles, your toes, the soles of your feet. Feel your feet, your toes, your soles on the carpet.

Sit down gently and give your 'great' body a big hug.

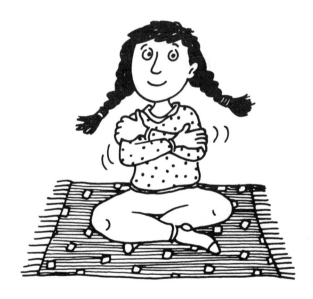

Discuss with the students what they have learnt about their bodies. Were there any surprises? What did they find out that was new? Again, ask them to share their thoughts, feelings and ideas.

Finish the activity by having a Body Quiz, making it quick and fun. Even older students quite enjoy this activity but you be the judge of this.

Body Quiz

Ask the students to stand up and make sure they have room to move.

Ask them to point to their head, ears, shoulders, etc. Finish by asking them to shake their whole wonderful bodies. Say:

Well done. You deserve a hug, so give yourself one ... and now be quiet and still for a moment.

5. Quiet Time

Students sit down slowly in their own space and are still for a minute. Put on the music tape and ask students to slowly and gently close their eyes and relax ... and listen to the music. Play the music quietly for 2–3 minutes.

Finishing Routine

I am going to count to 10. When I start counting, I want you to bring your thoughts back to this room, gently move your fingers and toes and slowly open your eyes. Eyes should be open by the time I reach 5. 1...2...3...4...5. Now as I count to 10 I want you to slowly, slowly sit up so that when I reach 10 we will all be sitting up. 6...7...8 (etc.) Well done. Now let's stand up and gently give our bodies a stretch. On tip toes, reach to the ceiling, stretch ... stretch.

Now lower your feet to the floor. That's great.

6. Reflection Time

Direct students back to the Working Circle for the discussion.

Discussion Points

- Body parts that were unfamiliar.
- The amazing things that our bodies can do. General discussion about how wonderful our bodies are: skin, feet, heart, brain. This discussion can form the basis of whole assignments, as suits the age and ability of your group. However, the main point to reinforce is that we must treat our bodies gently and with respect.
- Give positive feedback to students about how they worked in the session.
- Briefly revise the two concepts of body harmony and one's own space.

Practice Points

Ask students to:

- explain to the family what 'relax' means and the concepts of body harmony and one's own space;
- continue the quiet time each day;
- include a family member in their quiet time each day;
- have a body quiz with the whole family;
- remind themselves to treat their bodies gently each day, and to give themselves a hug often.

- Suggest students begin to work through pages 1 to 9 of their workbooks.

Closure

Play the music quietly, and direct the students to sit quietly, with their eyes closed, and think over what they have done in the session. After about 60 seconds, inform them that it's time to finish and leave the group. The students then open their eyes, stand up slowly, and quietly leave the room.

Classroom Activities

Ask students to:

- make posters such as 'Treat Your Body Gently', or 'I Have a Wonderful Body';
- put the names of the body parts in alphabetical order;
- make a list of words to describe their bodies and each part, for example, long legs, knobbly knees, soft hands;
- measure their bodies;
- compare hands, feet, arms, legs, finger sizes;
- make a chart of body sizes.

With them:

- play 'Simon Says'.

SESSION THREE

Aim
- to create awareness of our muscles and how we can make them tight or floppy.

Teaching Aids
cassette recorder, music tape, Overheads 7 and 8, overhead projector.

Vocabulary
muscles, tight, floppy.

Knowledge/Techniques
tightening and relaxing muscles.

1. Joining Together
Form the Working Circle allowing students time to quieten down and clear their minds of the day's activities.

2. Review Time
Body Awareness: By doing a quick body quiz, focus on those parts students had difficulty with last time. These might be waist, abdomen, thighs, shins, ankles, heart, elbows, bottom.

    N.B. Stress that our bodies should be treated gently.

3. & 4. Instruction and Practice Time

Introduction to Muscle Awareness
Show Overhead 7, explaining that knowing about our muscles is a step towards body harmony.

Show Overhead 8 and accompany it with an explanation of the muscles. This will vary according to the age of the students. For middle primary students, use a version of the following:

Muscles help many parts of our body to move. There are muscles we move ourselves and there are many more that move without us thinking about them. These do a special job inside our bodies, for example, there are muscles that keep our heart beating. Muscles are made up of bundles of fibres that stretch out flat when they are relaxed and bunch up tight, or contract, when they are being used. Muscles contain nerve cells and small blood vessels which give them the oxygen they need to do their work. If we hold our muscles tight for a long period of time, they 'jam up' or become knotted, and this sometimes causes pain messages to register in our brain. When we want to relax, we need to be able to check that our muscles are not tense and are not making our bodies tight.

OH 7

Body Harmony

MUSCLE KNOWLEDGE

- knowing the large muscle groups and working with them;

- recognizing your **'ouch'** spots and learning how to let them go, so you can be **calm** and **peaceful**.

OH 8

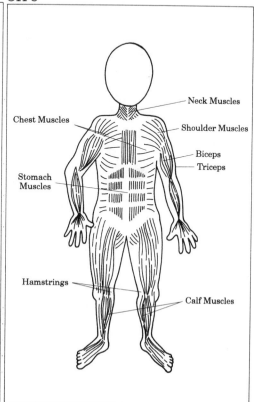

Neck Muscles

Chest Muscles

Shoulder Muscles

Biceps

Triceps

Stomach Muscles

Hamstrings

Calf Muscles

Muscle Exercises

(i) Now direct students to stand in their own space, keeping their eyes open if they prefer. Begin with:

Now, we are going to use our muscles to move our bodies in different ways. Remember, don't force movements.

And then using as much expression in your voice as you can:

Now, I want you to be, or make yourself into:
a tall, tall, strong and firm tree;
a floppy, floppy rag doll;
a long, long straight flag pole;
a wobbly, wobbly puppet;
a straight ... traffic light;
a tight ... spring;
a loose, loose overcoat;

a stiff ... fence post;
a wobbly, wobbly jelly fish;
a floppy ... flag;
a quiet, quiet mouse.

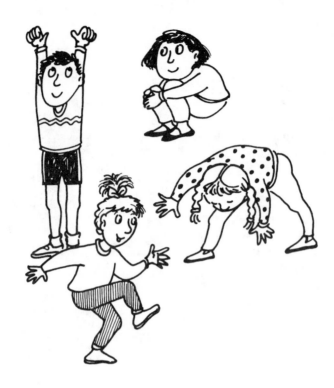

You may add to these similes as you wish, but end with a 'quiet, quiet, mouse'. At the end of the exercise, ask the students to sit down gently and be quiet.

Discuss with the students how their bodies felt being the various objects in the exercise. For example, were their bodies tight or floppy when they were a tall, tall tree, etc.

(ii) Direct students to stand, sit or lie in their own space. (This will depend on the age of your students.) Say:

I want you now to make your body tight, now let it be floppy.

Repeat this 4 or 5 times ending with a floppy posture.

(iii) Students lie in their own space. Say:

I want you now to close your eyes gently, then scrunch them up. Now slowly release them, but keep them gently closed. Now clench your teeth. Gently relax them. Now tighten your shoulders and chest. Now let them go, let them go floppy.

Continue the exercise with arms, hands, fingers, tummy and bottom, legs, feet, toes, whole body.

5. Quiet Time

Tell students that they will now begin quiet time and 'With your body floppy, let us listen to the music and relax'.

Play music for 3–4 minutes. Use the finishing routine to end the quiet time.

6. Reflection Time

Direct students back to the Working Circle.

Discussion Points

· Ask the students if they are aware that they have been practising a skill in using their muscles. Emphasize that this skill is essential in developing body harmony.

· How did the exercise feel for them? What did they learn to do with their muscles?

· What is the connection between relaxing and knowing about our muscles?

· How did the students feel when they made the different shapes?

Practice Points

· At intervals check whether the major muscle groups feel tight or floppy.

· Ask the children to check their muscles after they get into bed each night — are they tight or floppy?

· Continue a 'Quiet Time' each day.

Closure

As for previous session.

Classroom Activities

Ask students to:

· make a blank body shape and mark in the major muscle groups;

· make an extended list of similes;

· make a list of 'tight' and 'floppy' words;

· draw a person with tight muscles and floppy muscles;

· practise the skill of tightening muscles and letting them go, especially before beginning a quiet activity, for example, watching T.V. or listening to a story.

SESSION FOUR

Aims
- to extend the work we have done on muscles;
- to introduce the concept of 'ouch' spots.

Teaching Aids
cassette recorder, music tapes, Overheads 3 and 8.

Vocabulary
ouch, body scan.

Knowledge/Techniques
systematic relaxing of muscles, locating and being aware of 'ouch' spots.

1. Joining Together
Form the Working Circle allowing students time to quieten down and clear their minds of the day's activities.

2. Review Time

Muscles
Review what the muscles do, that is, to assist our bodies to move and to keep many important organs moving. (Use Overhead 8.) Look at those muscles we can direct to move and those muscles that move all the time without our even thinking about them. Ask what happens to our muscles when we relax them.

Recall last session's exercises when students made their bodies into various shapes and repeat the activity making different shapes.

3. & 4. Instruction and Practice Time

Introduction to 'ouch' spots
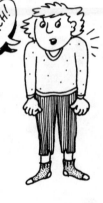

Discuss with the students what it feels like to hold their body muscles tightly. Ask them what is happening to their bodies when they do this.

Introduce the idea that when our muscles are held tightly for a long time, they begin to say 'ouch', because they are tight. Extend this idea to illustrate that at times when we feel frightened, excited, angry or anxious, we hold certain muscles tightly, and if we do this often, our muscles will begin to say 'ouch', like they did when we made tight shapes. We can call these 'ouch' spots. Stress that it is helpful to get to know where our 'ouch' spots are and when a muscle is saying 'ouch'.

Ask students to think about when they might have an 'ouch' spot and discuss which muscles may be saying 'ouch' and why. Ask the students to run a 'body scan', that is, a check to see if any of their muscles are saying 'ouch'.

Use Overheads 3 and 8 to identify 'ouch' spots.

Activity: Systematic Relaxation of Muscles

Introduce this activity by saying:

One good way to check for 'ouch' spots is to think about parts of your body and relax each muscle group. That way we get to know how muscles feel when they say 'ouch' and when they are relaxed. In the following exercise we are going to systematically relax the major parts of our body.

Direct students to sit in their own space, legs out in front, with hands resting on knees or by their sides. If they are a small group, they may sit in a circle, facing outwards. Check that they are comfortable and that none of their muscles are tight. **N.B.** Repeat each exercise twice.

Eyes:

Gently and slowly close them; now screw or scrunch them up, hold, and let them go. Let them go loose and floppy. Relax them.

Mouth and Cheeks:

Press your lips together firmly, hold, then let them go. Let them go loose and floppy. Relax them. Keeping your lips closed, push your mouth and cheeks out into a smile, hold, let them go. Let them go loose and floppy. Relax them. With your lips closed, push your mouth and lips forward, hold, then let them go. Let them go loose and floppy. Relax them.

Shoulders, Neck and Chest:

Push your shoulders up to your ears and hold your neck tight. Hold, then let them go. Let them go loose and floppy. Relax them. With your arms by your sides, push your shoulders back and hold the arms stiff. Hold, then let them go loose and floppy. Relax them.

Arms, Hands and Fingers:

With your arms by your sides, push them down and tighten the hands and fingers. Hold, then let them go. Let them go loose and floppy. Relax them.

Abdomen, Tummy and Bottom:

Pull them in tight and hold. Now let them go. Let them go loose and floppy. Relax them.

Thighs, Legs, Feet and Toes:

Hold your thighs, legs and feet tight and curl your toes under. Hold, then let them go loose and floppy. Relax them.

Whole Body:

Tighten it. Hold. Now let it go loose and floppy. Relax your whole body. Sit quietly and enjoy your body feeling loose and floppy and relaxed.

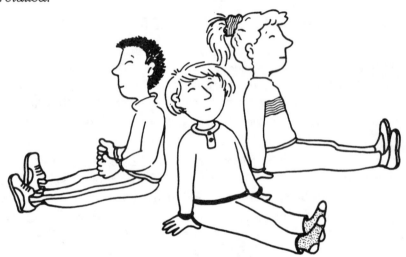

Activity: Loosening Up Muscles

Direct students to stand up slowly and to go gently into their own space. Repeat each exercise *five* times.

Head:

Very gently nod your head backwards and forwards. Now move it gently from side to side. Roll your head around and pretend you are using your head to follow the hands of the clock. Slowly, gently, move it around and around. Now, roll it back the other way, slowly and gently.

Shoulders:

Gently, raise your right shoulder as I count. 1...up. 2...down. Now your left shoulder. 1...up. 2...down. Now both shoulders. 1...up. 2...down. Roll your shoulders forward, then roll them backwards, then forward and backwards again.

Arms:

Stretch out your right arm in front of you at shoulder height and slowly and gently bend the arm, bringing your hand in to touch your shoulder. Repeat the same action with your left arm, then with both arms. Drop your arms and let them go loose and floppy. Gently give your arms a shake.

Tummy, Waist and Abdomen:

Stand with your feet a little apart. Now, think about where your abdomen, waist and tummy are. Now, gently lift your shoulders and with a sigh, drop them, sending the sigh into your abdomen, waist and tummy. Slouch a little.

Legs and Feet:

Gently put your hands on your hips. Lift one leg and give your leg and foot a shake. Repeat with the other leg and foot. Shake them gently. Swing first one leg, then the other, backwards and forwards, very slowly and gently.

Whole Body:

Just let it go loose and floppy, loose and floppy. Stand quite still for a moment and check that no part of your body is saying 'ouch'.

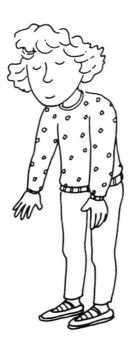

5. Quiet Time

With students remaining in their own space, put on the music. Allow about two minutes, then turn the music down and ask students to take their minds into their scalp, forehead, cheeks, jaw, mouth and eyes. Are any of these saying 'ouch'? Then say:

> *Slowly, let any tightness go and relax scalp, forehead, cheeks, jaw, mouth, eyes. Relax them.*
>
> *Take your mind into your neck, shoulders, arms, hands, fingers. Are any of these saying 'ouch'? Slowly let the tightness go. Relax neck, arms, hands, fingers. Relax them. Relax.*
>
> *Take your mind into your chest, your abdomen, tummy, bottom, thighs, legs, feet and toes. Are any of these saying 'ouch'? Slowly let the tightness go. Relax. Relax.*
>
> *Let your whole body relax and listen to the music.*

Turn the music up and let it play for about two minutes.

Use the finishing routine to end the quiet time.

6. Reflection Time

Direct students back to the Working Circle.

Discussion Points

- Give the students feedback about their work in this session. Ask them to recall which muscles were easy to relax and which were hard.
- Do they understand what a body scan is?
- Discuss those times when they are likely to get 'ouch' spots and which parts of their bodies the students think will be first to say 'Ouch, I'm tight!'.
- What can they do when this happens?

Practice Points

- Monitor 'ouch' spots, by reminding the children to check their bodies while in different activities, for example watching T.V., standing in line, listening to a story.
- Set homework for the class, by asking them to tell the family about 'ouch' spots and find out where other members of the family have them.
- Children continue to have their quiet time each day.
- Suggest children complete pages 10, 11 and 12 of their workbooks.

Closure

As for previous sessions.

Classroom Activities

Ask students to:
- draw their body and mark in their 'ouch' spots;
- trace a full size body. Students write their particular 'ouch' spots on cards and paste these on the body.
- make a bar graph of 'ouch' spots. Which 'ouch' spots are the most common?
- make a list of times when parts of their body say 'ouch';
- survey their family/class/friends to find out what 'ouch' spots they have.

- Include the muscle exercises as part of your everyday class activities. Shoulder, head and swinging arms exercises are particularly good.

SESSION FIVE

Aims

- to introduce the children to stretching techniques;
- to introduce the children to simple breathing techniques;
- to give the children practice in these techniques.

Teaching Aids

cassette recorder, music tape, Overheads 9 and 10.

Vocabulary

expand, contract, diaphragm, trachea, rib-cage, abdomen, inhale, exhale.

Knowledge/Techniques

stretching routines, understanding how we breathe, learning slow, deep and 'relax' breathing.

1. Joining Together

Form the Working Circle and allow time for students to quieten down and clear their minds of the day's activities.

2. Review Time

Review in the following way:

So far we have learnt three very important things which we need to know to be able to get our whole body to be calm and peaceful. We have learnt about the concept of body harmony. We have learnt about the concept of our own space and how to create our own physical, hearing, seeing and mind space. We have learnt how to work with our muscles, to check for 'ouch' spots, and how to make our large muscle groups loose and floppy. (Use Overheads 1–8 if helpful.)

Discuss homework and enquire how it went for the students.

3. & 4. Instruction and Practice Time

Introduction to Stretching Techniques

Reaching Stretches

Introduce these exercises by saying:

This is an extension of the muscle work that we have been doing over the last few weeks. It is also an activity that will help us to loosen our bodies.

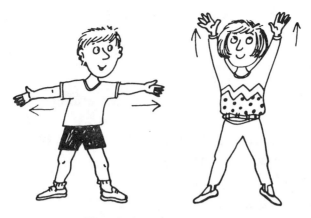

Reaching Stretches

i) Stretching Upwards: Direct students to stand with their feet a few centimetres apart, arms extended above the head, fingers spread. Feet remain on the floor. Ask them to imagine that they are trying to reach up to the ceiling, out through the ceiling and up to the sky.

With the feet apart, arms raised and fingers spread, stretch up, up, up as far as you can go. Hold. Let go and relax. Now repeat, seeing if you can stretch a little further. Repeat once more.

ii) Stretching Sideways: Feet will be positioned as before, with arms and fingers extended to the side of the body. Ask students to imagine that they are trying to reach out to the walls and beyond.

Start the stretch, feet apart, arms out, fingers spread, stretching out, out, out, to the walls as far as you can go. Hold. Let it go and relax.

Repeat the exercise twice more encouraging the students to reach out a little further at each stretch.

iii) Stretching Out in Front:

With feet a few centimetres apart, extend fingers, hands and arms out to the front, at shoulder height. Start the stretch, reaching far, far into the distance. Hold the stretch. Now let it go.

Repeat twice, encouraging the students to reach out a little further at each stretch.

iv) Stretching Down: Direct students to stand with feet a few centimetres apart, tummy and bottom held in, fingers, hands, arms, stretching down. Then:

Bend gently from the waist, reaching down through the floor, right down into the ground. Stretch down, down, down. Hold. Now let it go.

Repeat the exercise twice, encouraging them to reach down a little further with each stretch. At the end of the exercise, the students give their bodies a little shake, then sit quietly and gently in their own space, facing the teacher.

Breathing

Show Overhead 9 emphasizing that knowing about our breathing, different ways we can breathe, and controlling our breathing, like muscle knowledge, is another step towards body harmony.

Explanation of How We Breathe: (Use Overhead 10). The following explanation is suited to Grades 2–6.

OH 9   OH 10

Body Harmony # BREATHING · knowing how we breathe and controlling our breathing; · learning different types of breathing which will help us to be **calm** and **peaceful**.	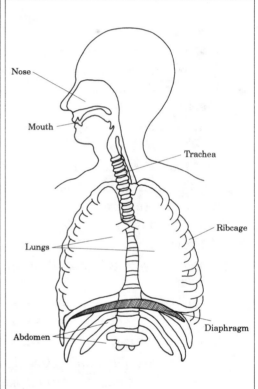

To have a healthy body, we need to be able to increase the amount of oxygen which our body gets. During our daily activities, the amount of oxygen we breathe in usually fills our lungs to only one-third of their capacity. If we learn to breathe slowly and deeply, we can not only increase our oxygen intake but also purify and revital-ize our bodies.

In order to relax, it is important to learn to control the way we breathe. In particular, we need to learn to slow our breathing, by breathing deeply . The main parts of our body that we use to breathe are: our nose, mouth, trachea, our lungs and two groups of muscles.

(Use the overhead to illustrate the position and function of these two groups of muscles.)

The first group is connected to our rib cage, and the other consists of a large sheet of muscles called the diaphragm which separates the chest space from the abdomen. When we breathe in through our nose or our mouth — this is called 'inhaling' — the air then goes down our trachea into our lungs. These expand when we inhale and bring in the air. They then contract, as we exhale and push air out of our lungs.

Our lungs are like a balloon, with the trachea being like the neck. The sheet muscles, known as our diaphragm, act as a pump, which moves up and down, creating pressure on the lungs to take air in — inhale — and send air out — exhale. The muscles attached to our rib-cage also help it to expand and contract.

These will be the parts of the body that we will be working with today.

Breathing Exercises

Introduce the breathing exercises with the following explanation:

The exercises we are going to do now will help our bodies to become calm and peaceful. We are going to observe our breathing, and observe how our muscles and the inside parts of our bodies work. When we learn to relax, we can actually slow our breathing and this helps to slow our heart rate, and then, our whole body. The exercises we learn today will help us to control our breathing.

i) **Observing Our Own Breathing:** Students sit in their own space, eyes open. Ask them to observe their breathing carefully. Are they breathing through their nose or mouth? Is their breathing slow or fast? As students breathe in through the nose, with their mouth closed, say to them, 'You are sending air through your trachea and into your lungs. Now breathe out through your nose'. Repeat three times.

ii) **Observing Our Inside Parts Working As We Breathe:** Tell students:

Place your hands lightly on your waist and move them slowly up until you reach your rib-cage. Rest your fingers gently on the edge of your rib-cage and be very still and quiet. Feel your muscles working. Feel the gentle up and down movement. (Take time to help students to do this. Ask them to feel what is happening when we breathe in and out.) *Notice the diaphragm as it contracts and expands. Next gently place your hands just above your chest and again be very still and quiet. Feel your breathing. It should be quiet, steady, even.*

Preparation for Breathing Exercises

Direct students to stand up, legs about 10 cms apart .

Stand on your toes and lift your hands over your head, gently moving up and down on the toes. Stretch and reach for the ceiling. Lower your heels and then loosely swing your arms around your body. You are now ready to learn to control your breathing.

iii) 'Relax' Breathing: Students sit in their own space, with their eyes closed. Legs are straight out in front of the body, with the hands on thighs. The students breathe in and out slowly through their nose. Then say:

We are now going to inhale through our nose while I count to 4. Hold your breath for 4 seconds, then breathe out saying the word R...E...L...A...X silently finishing by the time you reach 'X'. Repeat, lengthening the word, 'relax'. Repeat five times, each time lengthening the word. Let your breathing return to normal, open your eyes, and gently move your head and shoulders.

iv) Slow Breathing: Students lie in their own space in a relaxed position checking their bodies for tight spots.

Breathe in slowly to the count of 1, 2, 3. Hold for 1, 2, 3. Exhale to the count of 1, 2, 3. Rest 1, 2, 3.

Repeat, increasing the count by one each time. Breathing eventually should go to 10, depending on your group. Be guided by them.

v) Deep Breathing: The students lie in their own space, relaxed, with no tight spots. Explain to them that they are going to breathe slowly and deeply.

Breathe in, inhale, and send your breath deep down to your toes. Exhale and send your breath up from your toes and out slowly. Repeat five times.

5. Quiet Time

Continue the slow deep breathing to music. Allow about two minutes. Use the following finishing routine to bring the students out of the state of relaxation.

I want you now to start breathing normally. Go through your body and check each part: head, neck, shoulders, chest, arms, hands, tummy, etc. Now, roll slowly onto your left side and stretch. Now, roll onto your right side and stretch. When you are ready, begin to sit up. I will slowly count to 5, by which time you should be sitting up. 1...2...3...4...5. Now, as I count to 10 slowly stand up. 6...7...8...9...10.

6. Reflection Time

Direct students back to the Working Circle.

Discussion Points

- Give students feedback about their performance.
- Revise the anatomy details that were introduced.
- Reinforce the connection of breath control with the concept of body harmony.
- Discuss some of the situations when the children may wish to control their breathing. What happens when we become frightened, excited, angry, overtired or anxious?
- Discuss with the group the purpose, in evolution, for their physiological reaction and compare this reaction with situations they encounter.

Practice Points

- Find a few free minutes to practise stretching and breathing.
- Ask the students to teach their family or friends what they have learnt, and then discuss with them how that went.
- Brainstorm when and how they can practise these techniques, for example, in bed, on rising in the morning.

Closure

As for previous sessions.

Classroom Activities

Ask students to:

- make a chart to show what the class has learned, for example, body harmony, one's own space, working with muscles;
- research the origins of the human response to situations when we are frightened, anxious, excited, etc.;
- brainstorm situations when we need to slow our breathing;
- add new vocabulary words to word lists or personal dictionary;
- experiment with a balloon to show how our lungs work;
- brainstorm different imagery for the stretching exercises.

SESSION SIX

Aim
- to extend the work on breathing.

Teaching Aids
cassette recorder, music tape, Overheads 9 and 10.

Vocabulary
energy, refresh.

Knowledge/Techniques
extension of stretching and breathing skills.

1. Joining Together
Form the Working Circle allowing students time to quieten down and clear their minds of the day's activities.

2. Review Time
- Using Overhead 9, review the role of breathing in creating body harmony.
- Discuss practice points from the previous session.
- Using Overhead 10 go over the main body parts that we use in breathing: nose, mouth, trachea, lungs, rib-cage, diaphragm.
- Discuss the occasions when it is very useful to control the way we breathe.
- Recall the Relax and Slow breathing exercises from the last session and take students through each breathing routine once.

3. & 4. Instruction and Practice Time

Climbing Stretch Activity
Tell students that the following exercises are an extension of their muscle work. Stretching is a way of releasing tension in our bodies and letting go of 'ouch' spots so we are ready to relax. With each exercise the children are to imagine that they are climbing up and out of their bodies.

i) Direct students to stand with their legs about 10 cm apart, arms loosely by their sides. Ensure that they are relaxed in this position. Then:

Extend your arms out in front, at shoulder height, with your fin-

gers spread. Push your right arm up and out from the shoulder in a lifting, rolling movement. Now do this with the left arm. Imagine you are trying to climb out of quicksand. Alternate your arms five times.

ii) Students stand with their legs about 10 cm apart, arms, hands and fingers extended to the side, at shoulder height. They push up and out in a rolling action to the right side, then to the left. Encourage them to lean into the action and to imagine they are climbing out to each side. Repeat five times.

iii) Students stand on their toes, with legs about 10 cm apart. Arms, hands, fingers are extended above their heads. They reach up and roll out of their shoulders imagining that they are climbing up and out of their bodies, first to the right, then to the left. Repeat five times.

iv) Students sit on the floor, with legs outstretched in front. Arms, hands, fingers are extended at shoulder height in front. They roll shoulders, waist and hips in a climbing motion reaching out to the front, then to the right, then to the left. Repeat five times.

Breathing Exercises

Introduce these by saying:

Today, we are going to do breathing exercises. First, we will do cleansing breathing followed by a breathing experiment. Then we will practise our deep breathing which we learnt last week, before learning about energy breathing which helps to revitalize our bodies.

Cleansing Breathing

Explanation:

This breathing is used to get stale air out of our lungs, and thus clean them out. It is a very good breathing exercise to do when you get up in the morning. It is also good to do if you are tired, or have been working for a long period.

Direct students to stand in their own space, with legs shoulder-width apart, hands at sides.

Bend from the waist and take your arms to the floor, and as you do, slowly breathe out, emptying your lungs of all stale air. When your arms are at the floor, and your lungs are empty, cross over your arms and come up, breathing in slowly and bringing your arms up in a circle till they are above your head while I count from 1 to 7. Now as I count from 1 to 4, I want you to bring your arms down to your sides, pushing your breath out slowly through your mouth until your arms touch your sides. Wait 1 or 2 seconds.

Repeat the exercise five times, then congratulate the students on getting rid of the stale air from their bodies.

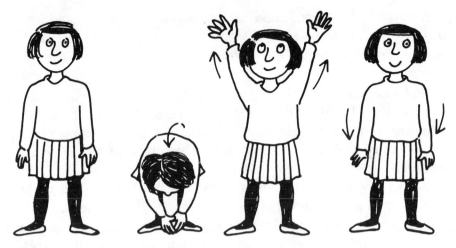

Cleansing Breathing

Breathing Experiment

Begin with an explanation:

This is a little experiment to show how our heart rate and our breathing are related. Place your hands on your chest, and feel your breathing. (Allow about a minute.) Now, jog slowly on the spot for two minutes, not quickly, but steadily. Now, place your hands on your chest again to feel your breathing. Listen to it.

Discuss the difference in breathing and heart rate, and talk about those times when the heart rate increases, for example, when one is scared, angry or exercising.

Review: Deep Breathing

Introduce this exercise by telling students that it will deliberately slow down their breathing. Direct them to stand in their own space, with feet slightly apart.

Inhale slowly, seeing, in your mind's eye, your breath as it comes into your body. Send it right down to your toes, pushing it down, down through your body to your toes. Now, slowly let the breath come up, up from your toes to exhale through your mouth.

Repeat the exercise eight times, counting aloud for the students from 1 to 5 while they inhale and 5 to 10 while they exhale. Then ask the students to place their hands on their chests again, to listen to and feel their breathing.

Discuss with them: What has happened to their bodies? How do they feel now?

Energy Breathing

This breathing helps us to recharge our bodies and minds after exercise or long periods of work.

Direct the students to lie in their own space and to relax, checking for tight spots. Ask them to concentrate on their breathing for thirty seconds. Then say:

Imagine, now, that your breath is golden energy, like a bright golden light. This will recharge your bodies. Slowly breathe in, and take the golden energy down through your body. Send it into each part of your body: arms, fingers, chest, legs, feet, toes. Flood your body with the golden energy. Breathe out slowly and take the stale air out, pushing it out of your body ... out through the top of your head.

Repeat this exercise five times, taking the children through it each time.

5. Quiet Time

The children continue with the breathing, while you play music for three to four minutes. Use the finishing routine to bring students out of relaxation.

6. Reflection Time

Discussion Points

· Give the students feedback about their work.
· Revise the types of breathing exercises done in the session:
  – cleansing breathing to clean out the lungs;
  – deep breathing, to slow down the breathing rate;
  – energy breathing to refresh the body and give it energy.
· Discuss the breathing experiment. Was it easy to slow down the breathing?
· Discuss the energy breathing. How did it feel? When might it be helpful?

Practice Points

· Ask the students to practise the stretching and cleansing breathing in the morning, and deep breathing at night, at home.
· Encourage the students to use energy breathing when they have been sitting working for extended periods of time.
· Suggest they complete page 13 of their workbooks.

Closure

As for previous sessions.

Classroom Activities

· Students illustrate one of the breathing exercises from this session.
· Teach students about the pulse, and how to record it.
· Do climbing and stretching exercises as a break between activities.

- Students draw the body, or provide an outline of the body, on which they mark the places where the pulse can be felt.
- Try a class experiment with students charting their pulse at rest, and while jogging. Encourage students to repeat the experiment with their family
- Students illustrate some situations when the heart rate will increase.
- Stretch with your class first thing in the morning and combine this with cleansing breathing.

SESSION SEVEN

Aims
· to introduce the concept of using our brain to create pictures in our mind;
· to help students to use this skill to assist them in imagery exercises.

Teaching Aids
cassette recorder, music tape, Overheads 11 and 12.

Vocabulary
imagery, brain, complicated, physical, imagination.

Knowledge/Techniques
'Brick Wall' stretching, breathing exercises, imagery exercises.

1. Joining Together
Form the Working Circle and allow students time to quieten down and clear their minds of the day's activities.

2. Review Time
With the group, go over the four important concepts that help them relax: knowledge of body parts, inside and out; creating one's own space; working with muscles; controlling breathing.

Discuss the last session and the practice they did.

3. & 4. Instruction and Practice Time
Brick Wall Stretch
Introduction: Remind students that they have learnt that stretching is a good way of letting go of muscle tension and 'ouch' spots and of working the muscles. Today they will learn another stretching exercise called Brick Wall Stretching in which they imagine they are trying to push over a big brick wall. So, each stretch needs to be a very strong one. Direct students to stand with feet firmly planted on the floor about 10 cm apart.

i) Front Stretch:

Stand with your arms at shoulder height, hands bent up from the wrist, fingers straight and together. Now imagine that there is a big, red brick wall in front of you. Really see the wall in your mind. Now, stretch out your arms and push the wall ... push ... push ... push the wall. Now relax, dropping your arms to your sides. Repeat this exercise five times, relaxing after each stretch.

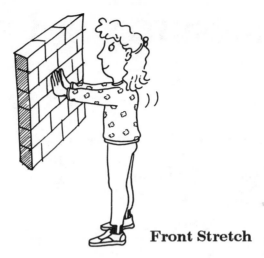

Front Stretch

ii) Upwards Stretch:

Imagine the brick wall is now above your head. With your arms and hands above your head, push against the brick wall. Try to push the wall away. Stretch up, up, up and push the wall away. Relax, with your arms dropping loosely. Repeat five times, relaxing after each stretch.

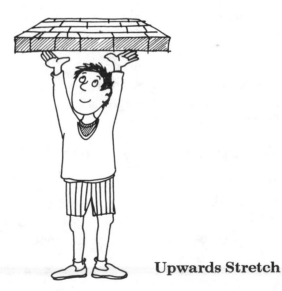

Upwards Stretch

iii) Side Stretch:

The big, red brick wall is now on your left side and I want you to turn from the waist to push against it. With both arms out at shoulder height, and hands bent upwards, turn your head, shoulders and arms to the left, and stretch out ... out, to push over the wall. Relax, then turn to the right and repeat the action. Alternate left and right, repeating each stretch five times, and relaxing between each stretch. Finish with a gentle stretch.

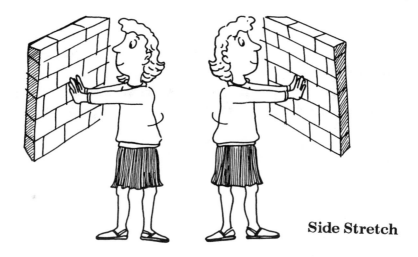

Side Stretch

Review: Cleansing Breathing

Stand in your own space, with your legs about 10 cm apart, hands at your sides. Bend from your waist and take your arms to the floor, slowly breathing out deeply. Hold. Now, while I count to 6 I want you to cross over your arms at floor level and come up, bringing your arms up in a circle above your head. 1...2...3...4. Pause for 2 seconds and then repeat. Repeat four or five times.

Introduction to the Concept of Imagery

Explanation: How images assist with relaxation. (Use Overheads 11, 12, 13). Discuss with the group how wonderful their bodies are and the way the body's various systems, such as breathing and the digestive system, work. Review how they have been working with their bodies over the past sessions, reinforcing the concept of body harmony. Discuss the function of the brain, using Overhead 13 and the script below.

Today, we are going to talk about our brain and how it can help us to relax.

Our brain controls our body's functions — our heart's beating, our lungs breathing, our digestion — even while we are asleep.

Our brain helps us to make sense of the world around us. We perceive the world around us through our five senses — hearing, sight, smell, touch and taste — which send messages along the nerves to the brain. Our brain's memory enables us to recognize this information and make sense of the message.

In turn, the brain sends messages back along the nerves to our muscles so we can act. For example: you are crossing a road and your eyes see and your ears hear something. They send messages to your brain where the memory immediately works out that that 'something' is a car. Your brain works out what you need to do to

55

avoid being hit and sends a message along the nerves to your muscles to jump out of the way. This all happens in a split second.

Your brain also controls speech which enables you to communicate with the world around you.

We can use our brain to create pictures in our mind. (Show Overhead 11.) These pictures are called images. They are not real, only in our mind.

OH 11

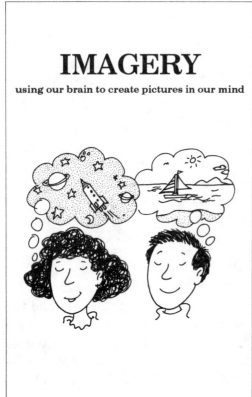

OH 13

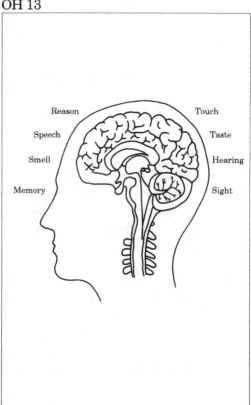

Remind the class that they already use images to help them in their breathing and stretching exercises, such as the energy breathing and brick wall exercises. Discuss how this skill of creating mental images may be valuable in their lives, for example, as a means of learning new or difficult things. Summarize using Overhead 12.

N.B. Stress that in using images or pictures, the children don't actually do any action or go anywhere, but they create the images themselves and do the actions in their mind.

OH 12

My Own Space

IMAGERY

using our brain to create pictures in our mind

These pictures can help us:

- to get our whole body to be **calm** and **peaceful**;

- to feel **great** about ourselves;

- to practise new or difficult things.

---

5. Quiet Time

Imagery Exercises

Direct students to find their own space and quietly lie in it. You may need to check that they are not in anyone else's space. Take the students through a check of their bodies for any tight spots. Go through each of their body parts — arms, hands, fingers, chest, abdomen, tummy, bottom, thighs, legs, feet — asking them to picture each part as you refer to it. Conclude by saying:

> *Relax ... relax ... relax, and let all the tightness go. Now, in your own space, listen to your breathing. Slow it down. Breathe in slowly, and send the breath down to fill out your lungs ... now, let it out slowly, slowly, slowly. Now, take three more slow breaths.*

Ask the students to clear their minds, and concentrate on your voice because they are now going to use their brains to make a very special picture. Remind them that they will not actually do anything, they will just see themselves performing that particular action in their mind. Now read, or say the following, slowly and quietly to the group:

57

I want you to think about the space you are in. Feel yourself in the quiet, quiet space. (Pause for about 5 seconds.) Now, I want you to build a wall right around your space. Make it a high wall. See that wall in your mind. Now I want you to put a secret door in your wall. No one else will know where that door is, just you. See that secret door in your mind. Paint that secret door in your favourite colour. (Pause for 5 seconds.)

Now, go through the door. Close it behind you. Look around your own space and see the wall and the door. Put something for you to lie on in that space, perhaps a bed, or a soft, cosy rug, or some soft smooth grass, or a fluffy white cloud. In your mind, feel what you are going to lie on. Now lie down gently. It is so, so, soft and comfortable. Let yourself sink down, down into its softness. Your whole body is light and soft, calm and peaceful, calm and peaceful.

Allow a minute for them to lie in this spot, then slowly turn down the music.

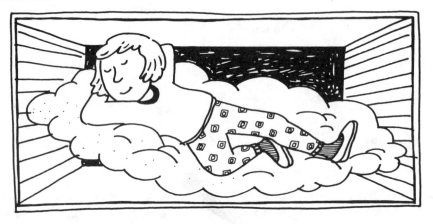

Now, end the quiet time with the following finishing routine:

Now, you are going to get ready to leave your comfortable, soft space. In your mind, I want you to get up from your soft, comfortable lying space and stretch your body again. Now, find your secret door, stand near your door and say good-bye to your space. (Pause for 5 seconds.) Slowly open the door and let yourself out and shut the door behind you. Now you are back in the room at (name the place). *Feel the carpet that you are lying on. Gently wiggle your fingers. Gently wiggle your toes. Stretch your body and relax. Roll onto your left side and stretch. Roll on to your right side and stretch. Now, as I begin to count, slowly begin to sit up. When I reach 5, you will be sitting up, with your eyes open ... 1...2...3...4...5. Stand up and stretch, up and up. Relax. Well done.*

6. Reflection Time

Discussion Points

- Give feedback to the children and ask them about the session. Which parts did they find enjoyable? Which difficult?
- What was their special place like?
- Brainstorm the occasions in which they could use imagery to help them and discuss which images they would choose.

Closure

As for previous sessions.

Classroom Activities

Ask students to:

- draw and/or write a description about their special place, and share it with a classmate;
- make graphs, for example, of the colours the students painted their secret doors, of what they were lying on;
- make a list of other images they could use for that week's stretching activity;
- draw illustrations of the stretching exercises.
- Practise daily with the children creating an image of their own special space.
- Be creative in using situations that arise in the day-to-day life of your class to practise using imagery.

SESSION EIGHT

Aim

· to continue and extend guided imagery skills.

Teaching Aids

cassette recorder, music tape, Overheads 11–14.

Vocabulary

no new words.

Knowledge/Techniques

extension of stretching, breathing exercises, review of key components of relaxation, extension of imagery skills.

1. Joining Together

Form the Working Circle and allow students time to quieten down and clear their minds of the day's activities.

OH 14

KEY CONCEPTS OF RELAXATION

Body Harmony:
Getting the inside and outside parts
of the body working together.

Skill Areas

· Body Knowledge	–	knowing the parts of our body and how they can work together;
· Muscle Knowledge	–	knowing the large muscle groups and working with them;
· Breathing	–	knowing how we breathe and controlling our breathing.

Our Own Space:
Being able to be in our own space.

Skill Areas

· Our Own Space	–	creating our own physical, seeing, hearing, mind space;
· Imagery	–	using our brain to create pictures in our mind.

2. Review Time

Discuss with the students what they did in the last session: using their brain to create pictures in their mind, that is, imagery. Revise the concepts behind this, using Overheads 11, 12, 13. Then show Overhead 14: the key concepts of relaxation.

3. & 4. Instruction and Practice Time

Stretching Exercises
Overhead Stretch:

Stand with feet 10 cm apart, hands by sides. Inhale slowly and deeply and raise your arms slowly above your head and stretch. Hold for the count of 3. Exhale slowly as you lower your arms and let them come to rest on your thighs. Repeat three times.

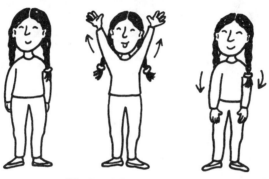

(i) Overhead Stretch

Side Stretch (1):

Now, stand with feet as before, and arms by your sides. Inhale slowly and turn your head and take a small step to the right, raising your right arm overhead and stretch. Your left arm slides down your leg a little. Your head lilts slightly to the left. Hold for a count of 3, exhale slowly, and lower your arm to your side. Turn your head to the left and repeat the exercise on that side. Alternate five times.

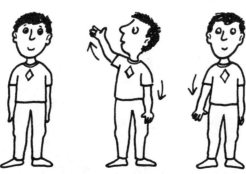

(ii) Side Stretch (1)

61

Back Stretch:

With your feet positioned as above, hands on thighs and body bent slightly forward, inhale deeply and raise your arms up and over your head. Stretch back just a little and hold for a count of 3. Exhale and slowly bring your arms forward and rest them on your thighs. Repeat three times.

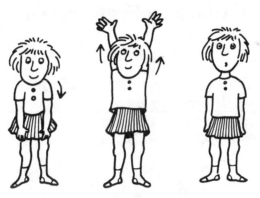

(iii) **Back Stretch**

Side Stretch (2):

With your feet as above, and your arms by your sides, inhale slowly and deeply and raise both arms up overhead. Let the backs of your hands touch above your head. Hold for 3 seconds. Exhale slowly and lower your arms to your sides. Repeat three times.

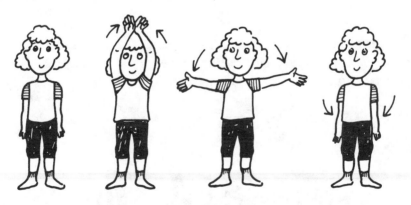

(iv) **Side Stretch (2)**

Body Circles: Ask students to stand in a relaxed position, feet a few centimetres apart. They, then, gently swing their arms around their bodies from the waist.

Breathing Exercise: 'Relax' Breathing

Direct students to sit in their own space in a relaxed and comfortable position, hands on thighs. Then:

Slowly inhale through your nose while I count to 4. 1...2...3...4. Hold for 5, 6. Exhale slowly as I count 7–10 saying in your own mind, R...E...L...A...X.

Repeat five times, counting aloud for the students each time.

5. Quiet Time

Imagery Exercise

Introduction: Discuss briefly with the students the skill of using the brain to make pictures in their mind. Stress that these pictures are images and that they can use them to relax and feel good about themselves. Then direct them to lie in their own space, checking that there are no tight spots. Begin the exercise:

Let any tightness go, and relax the muscles until they are floppy. Become aware of your breathing and begin to slow it down, by saying to yourself, 'Slowly in, slowly out, slowly in, slowly out'. Concentrate on my voice as you make pictures in your mind.

I want you to think of the space you are in. Feel yourself in this quiet space. Now build a wall around your space. See the wall in your mind. It is a high strong wall. (Pause 5 seconds.) Recall the secret door you put in your wall. It was painted in your favourite colour. See the door in your mind, and slowly open it and let yourself into your special space, making sure that you shut the door tightly.

Look around your space and find that special something you like to lie on: a bed, a soft rug, or maybe some smooth grass, some warm white sand, or soft feathers. Now lie down on it. (Pause 5 seconds.) In your mind, feel what you are lying on. It is so soft and comfortable. Let yourself sink into its softness, down, down into the softness. Your whole body becomes light and soft, calm and peaceful, calm and peaceful. (Pause 5 seconds.)

Today, there is a light breeze blowing. It gently blows your hair and touches your face. It is a cool, cool (or 'warm, warm' according to the season) breeze that is gentle and light. Feel it softly touching your hair and your face and gently blowing around your body, so that you are cool (warm), calm and peaceful. Your gentle, soft breeze has a wonderful smell. Take a deep breath and smell the breeze as it gently blows around you, making you cool (warm), calm and peaceful.

(**Note:** The type of breeze needs to fit the season in which you are running the session. For example, on a hot day, the breeze will be cool, with a fresh, clean smell like rain. Conversely, in the winter, the breeze will be warm, evoking sweet strong smells of a warm kitchen.)

Quietly switch on the music, and let the students remain quiet, listening to the music for about 2–3 minutes. Slowly turn the music down as you say:

Get ready now to leave your space and the gentle breeze. (Pause 5 seconds.) In your mind, I want you to stretch your body, and then relax it. I want you to leave your lying space, and stretch your body again. Find your secret door and slowly open it and let yourself out, shutting the door carefully behind you. (Pause 5 seconds.)

Use the following finishing routine to bring the children out of relaxation.

Now you are back in the room at ... (name the place). Feel the carpet you are lying on. Stretch your body. Relax it. Roll onto your left side and stretch. Roll onto your right side and stretch ... Well done. As I begin to count, slowly begin to sit up. When I reach 5, you will be sitting up with your eyes open. 1...2...3...4...5. Now stand up and relax.

6. Reflection Time

Discussion Points
· Give students individual feedback about how they worked during the session.
· How did they feel? What colours did they see? What smells did they smell? Did they feel cool, (or warm)?
· Discuss the calm and peaceful parts of their special place.

Practice Points
· Practise Relax breathing.
· Start each morning with a stretching exercise.
· Give each child the task of teaching someone at home a breathing or stretching exercise.

Closure
As for previous sessions.

Classroom Activities
Ask students to:
· paint a picture about the imagery in today's session;
· draw or write about their own special place, where they can go to relax and feel good about themselves;
· make a list of ideas that could make them feel cool or warm;
· design their own chart about the key components of relaxation.
· Find time each day to practise with the children getting into their own space.

SESSION NINE

Aims

- to extend guided imagery skills;
- to introduce a new relaxation technique: scalp massage.

Teaching Aids

cassette recorder, music tapes (music should have a floating tempo), Overhead 14.

Vocabulary

scalp, massage.

Knowledge/Techniques

revision of key concepts of relaxation, extension activities in stretching, breathing, muscles, and imagery, introduction of scalp massage.

1. Joining Together

Form the Working Circle allowing the students time to quieten down and clear their minds of the day's activities.

2. Review Time

Review the five key concepts of relaxation — use Overhead 14.

3. & 4. Instruction and Practice Time

Loosening-up Activities

Direct students to stand in their own space, feet a few centimetres apart. Each exercise is repeated five times.

i) Head:

Very gently, nod your head backwards and forwards. Now move it slowly from side to side. Roll your head around and pretend that you are using your head to follow the hands of the clock. Slowly, gently, move it around, and around. Now, roll it back the other way, slowly and gently.

ii) Shoulders:

Gently, lift each shoulder, one at a time, and let it drop. Lift your right shoulder, 1 ... up. 2 ... down. Now your left ... 1 ... 2. Now both ... 1 ... 2. Roll shoulders forward, then roll them backwards, then forward and backwards again.

iii) **Arms:**

Stretch out your right arm in front of you at shoulder height. Now, slowly bend it so that your hand touches your shoulder. Repeat five times. Now, lift your left arm in front of you, at shoulder height, and slowly bend it so that your hand touches your shoulder. Repeat five times. Extend both arms at shoulder height, then gently bend them so that your hands touch your shoulders. Repeat five times. Drop the arms and let them go loose and floppy. Gently give your arms a shake.

iv) **Tummy, Waist and Abdomen:**

Stand with your feet a little apart. Now think about where your abdomen, waist and tummy are. Gently lift your shoulders and with a sigh drop them down, sending the sigh into your abdomen, waist and tummy. Slouch a little. Repeat five times. Now turn your body from the waist. Let your arms swing gently and loosely to the left, to the right, to the left, to the right. Let your arms, tummy, and abdomen be floppy and loose. Repeat five times.

v) **Legs and Feet:**

Gently put your hands on your hips. Lift one leg and give your leg and your foot a shake. Now repeat with the other leg and foot. Shake them gently. Repeat five times. Swing your right leg slowly backwards and forwards, then the left leg backwards and forwards, very slowly and gently. Repeat five times.

vi) **Whole Body:**

Just let it go loose and floppy, loose and floppy. Stand quiet and still for a moment and check that no part of your body is saying 'ouch'.

Cleansing Breathing

Direct students to stand in their own space, with their legs about shoulder-width apart, hands at their sides.

Bend from the waist and take your arms to the floor, at the same time slowly breathing out, emptying your lungs of all stale air. When your arms are at floor level, and your lungs are empty, cross over arms and come up, while I count from 1 to 7. Inhale, bringing your arms up in a circle till they're above your head. 1...2...3...4... 5...6...7. Now, as I count from 1 to 4, bring your arms down to your sides, pushing your breath out slowly through your mouth until your arms touch your sides. 1...2...3...4. Wait 2 seconds. Repeat five times.

Scalp Massage

Introduction: Tell students that they are now going to learn a useful technique for getting rid of the tension we often have in our scalp. It's an activity they can also do with a friend or someone in their family.

Direct students to sit in their own space and to spend a few minutes feeling their scalp. Ask them to tell you how their scalps feel and if anyone feels any bumps on their scalp. Then they carefully place their hands over their ears, slowly moving their hands up to the head, until their fingers meet at the top of the head. Gently, but firmly, they move the fingers around the scalp, so that they feel all over the head, rather like washing the hair. Do this for 30 seconds. Then, ask them to lower their arms and place their hands in their laps and, then, to shake their hands gently.

This can be a difficult exercise, so you will have to demonstrate the massage, and give individual help to some students.

Repeat the activity. Depending on the maturity of the group, you may like to let them work in pairs giving each other a scalp massage.

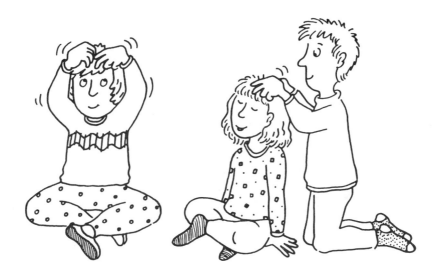

Scalp Massage

Muscle Exercise

Tell students that today they are going to do an exercise which will help them relax their muscles.

Direct students to lie in their own space, with enough room above their heads for their arms. Then:

Curl your toes over and tighten up all the muscles in your feet and legs, so they are very, very tight. Hold for 10 seconds. Now let the tightness go. Relax all the muscles.

Tighten the tummy, abdomen and bottom, so they are very, very tight. Hold for 10 seconds. Now let the tightness go. Relax.

Think about your back, chest, shoulders, arms, hands, and fingers. Gently stretch out your fingers. Now, tighten all the muscles in these parts of your body, so they are very, very tight. Hold for 10 seconds. Let the tightness go. Relax.

Now tighten your whole body. Gently stretch your hands up over your head. Tighten all the muscles, from the tips of your fingers to the end of your toes. Tighten ... tighten ... hold. Now let the tightness go. Relax, relax all your muscles. Stay in your space, breathing at your own rate and feel all your muscles relaxed. (Allow a minute.)

5. Quiet Time

Use music with a floating tempo for this activity. (See Part 5.) Have it turned down low as you begin speaking.

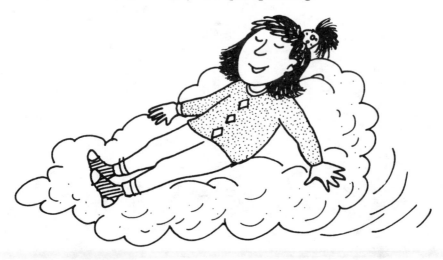

Guided Imagery

Today, I want each of you to use your brain to make pictures in your mind of your special space and I want you to put yourself in that special space. Remember ... your high, strong wall ... your secret door ... your special something to lie on. Now take yourself into your special space. (Allow 30 seconds.)

Now that you are in your special space in your mind, I want you to see large fluffy clouds up in the sky above you. There is one very special white fluffy cloud. Watch it as it slowly floats down to-

wards you and stops just near you. As it is a special cloud, you lie down on it. It is so softly comfortable that you sink down, down, into its wonderful softness. Slowly, your big white fluffy cloud gently begins to float up, up, up, into the sky ... Now, you are floating along on your cloud. You are so light and free and you gently, gently glide along. It is so quiet and peaceful. Rest now, and enjoy the wonderful peacefulness. (Slowly turn the music up and let the students relax for a minute. Gradually turn the music down.)

Now your cloud must leave you. It glides down and comes to rest in your special space. Slowly you step off it, and watch as it floats away, high up into the sky. (Pause for five seconds, then move into the following finishing routine.)

It is time for you also to leave your special space, so find your se-cret door, and let yourself out. Now you are back in the room at ... (name the place). *Feel the carpet you are lying on. Stretch your body and relax it. Roll onto your left side and stretch. Roll onto your right side and stretch. Now, as I begin to count, slowly begin to sit up. When I get to 5, sit up with your eyes open. Now stand and stretch up, up. Relax. Well done!*

6. Reflection Time

Discussion Points
- Which exercises do students prefer for stretching, breathing, muscles?
- When can they use these exercises?
- What did students think of the imagery exercise?

Practice Points
- Students do loosening-up exercise for head and shoulders while sitting, reading, doing written work, watching T.V.
- They practise the muscle exercise when they get into bed, working through the whole body until it is loose and floppy.
- They give someone at home a scalp massage.
- They teach someone in their family to give them a scalp massage.
- They complete pages 14 to 18 of their workbooks.

Closure
As for previous sessions.

Classroom Activities
Ask students to:
- observe different types of clouds. Record what they look like;
- write directions on and illustrate how to give a scalp massage;
- compile a word list to explain what it feels like to be relaxed.

SESSION TEN

Aim

- to extend guided imagery skills.

Teaching Aids

cassette recorder, music tapes, Certificates for students.

Vocabulary

no new vocabulary.

Knowledge/Techniques

extension of imagery skills.

1. Joining Together

Form the Working Circle allowing students time to quieten down and clear their minds of the day's activities.

2. Review Time

Brief discussion of how the practice went.

3. & 4. Instruction and Practice Time

Introduction: Tell students that in this segment of the session they are going to practise scalp massage and one muscle and one breathing exercise.

Scalp Massage

Direct students to their own space. Then:

Place your hands over your ears carefully, and then slowly move them up till your fingers meet at the top of your head. Gently, but firmly, move your fingers around so that you are feeling all over your scalp, taking away any tightness that is there. (Allow 30 seconds.) Lower your hands to your lap, then give your fingers and hands a little shake.

Muscle Exercise

Body scan for 'ouch' spots:

Now lie in your own space. Think about your main body parts and check that they are not saying 'Ouch! I'm tight'. If they are, let the tightness go. Start with your toes and feet and gradually move up your body, checking each main part. (Allow one minute.) Rest in your own space and let yourself be loose and floppy. (Allow 30 seconds of quiet time.)

Breathing Exercise

Ask students to choose one of the breathing exercises that they can do sitting in their own space. It may be 'Relax' breathing, Slow breathing, Energy breathing, or Deep breathing. Tell them to choose the one they would *like* to do, and just quietly think about how to do it. (Allow 10 seconds.)

Now begin your breathing exercise ... off you go, slowly and quietly, slowly and quietly. (Allow a minute for this exercise.) *Well done! Let your breathing go back to normal, and have another quiet time, lying in your own space.*

5. Quiet Time

Guided Imagery

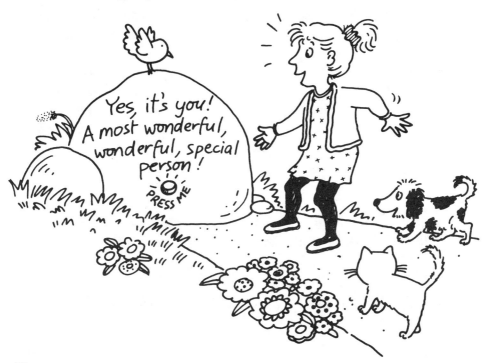

Have some music — quiet, peaceful with no sudden changes in tempo — ready to turn on, and begin the following:

Today, you are going to use your brain again to help you get into your special space, but one thing will be different. When you go into your special space, you will find a beautiful, thick, soft rug to lie on. It will be made of wonderful, soft wool in your favourite colour. Now, take yourself to your special place. (Allow 10 seconds.) *Close your door and gently lie down on your beautiful rug.* (Allow 5 seconds.)

Feel your rug underneath you. It is so soft, let yourself sink, sink into its wonderful softness. (Pause 5 seconds then turn the music on softly. This will provide a background for your voice.) *Your rug is turning into a magic carpet and it is slowly, slowly rising up over your wall, up up, into the sky. You are floating along on your magic carpet, gently, gently floating along, floating along.* (Pause 5 seconds.)

Down below, you notice that there is an island, and your carpet slowly, slowly begins to float down towards this island. Soon, it lands on soft green grass, and you lie still for a minute and breathe in the fresh, clean air. Listen to the sound of the birds in the trees and feel the gentle breeze blowing around you. It has a fresh, clean smell. (Pause 5 seconds.) *Slowly, get off your carpet and look around. It is such a beautiful island — the grass is very green and soft, the trees are tall and graceful; there are many beautiful flowers growing.*

Now you see a sandy pathway and you begin to follow it. As you go, you see all the wonderful and beautiful things on the island: the birds, flowers, trees, animals. (Pause for 5 seconds.) *You are nearly at the end of your path and ahead of you is a very, very large, flat rock which is standing up out of the grass. It looks like a giant T.V. screen. As you get nearer, you can see a big red button which is stuck on the bottom of the rock. Nearer and nearer you go and soon you see some writing underneath the button. It says 'PRESS ME'. Carefully you step toward the button and gently press it. You take some steps backwards so that you can see the whole front of the rock. Just then a big, big picture of you appears on the rock, and underneath is written this question, 'Do you know who this is?' Just as you open your mouth to answer, a message flashes up on the rock, saying 'Yes, it's you! A most wonderful, wonderful, special person!' All of a sudden, you feel very, very happy, so happy that you give yourself a big hug and say, 'Yes, I am a wonderful, wonderful, special person. I am wonderful and special!' and you really feel wonderful and special. Feel it now.* (Pause 5 seconds.)

Now, your image and the message are fading. They are gone and so is the red button. Slowly, you turn and go back down the path. You feel so light, peaceful and happy inside and repeat over and over, 'I am a wonderful and special person. I am a wonderful and special person!' (Pause 5 seconds.)

Now, you are back where you left your magic carpet, and you climb on board. Stretch out your wonderful and special body. Slowly, slowly, your carpet rises and begins to leave your beautiful island. Soon, you are high up above your island, which looks like a tiny spot. Whisper goodbye to your island and gently float along on your carpet. (Pause 5 seconds.)

Your carpet begins to float downwards again and very soon you find yourself back in your special place again. Slowly, you get up off your rug and give it a gentle shake. Now roll it up and find a special place where you carefully store it away. (Pause 5 seconds before beginning the following finishing routine.)

It is time to leave your special place now, so carefully let yourself out through your secret door. (Pause 5 seconds.) *Feel the carpet on which you are lying ... wriggle your fingers. Now your toes. Stretch your body and relax it. Roll onto your left side and stretch. Roll onto your right side and stretch. As I begin to count, slowly begin to sit up. When I get to 5, you will be sitting up with your eyes open. 1...2...3...4...5. Now, stand and stretch up and up and relax. Well done, you wonderful special people! Give yourselves a big, big hug.*

6. Reflection Time

Discussion and Practice Points

As this is the last session, the discussion will focus on reviewing the skills the students have learnt and a reminder that they can use their workbooks to help them remember and practise their relaxation skills.

7. Presentation of Certificates

This should be a formal segment, to increase its significance and reinforce the importance of the work the students have done over the weeks. Invite the parents and other significant people, for example, the Principal. When giving out the certificates, make some personal, encouraging statement to each student.

Classroom Activities

· Ask students to bring their workbooks to school and have them discuss them with a partner.
· Prepare a class relaxation quiz.
· With the class, prepare an information session on relaxation for the school assembly, newsletter, etc.
· Provide a school display about the program.

REFERENCES

Bernard, M. E. (1990), *Taking the Stress out of Teaching.* Collins Dove, Melbourne.

Garth, M. (1990), *Starbright: Meditations for Young Children.* Collins Dove, Melbourne.

Hendricks, G. and Wills, R. (1989), *The Centering Book: Awareness Activities for Children, Parents and Teachers.* Prentice Hall Press, Englewood Cliffs, NJ.

Hendricks, G. and Roberts, T. B. (1989), *The Second Centering Book.* Prentice Hall Press, Englewood Cliffs, NJ.

Hindley, J. and Rawson, C. (1975), *How Your Body Works.* Usborne Publishing, London.

Madders, J. (1987), *Relax and Be Happy: Techniques for 5–18 Year-Olds.* Unwin Paperbacks, London.

Montgomery, B. (1982), *Coping with Stress.* Pitman Health Information Series, Pitman, Melbourne.

Spielberger, C. (1979), *Understanding Stress and Anxiety.* Nelson, Florida.

Part Three

ACTIVITIES FOR SHORT ROUTINES

Stretching Exercises

These exercises are used as a 'refresher' or 'waking up' for the body at any time throughout the school day. They are also an excellent way of revitalizing tired or stiff muscles. Visual images have been suggested, but you might need to vary these for your particular age group.

The exercises may also be varied by doing them lying down. In this position, the children can spread out and stretch down through the feet and toes and up through the arms, hands and fingers.

Reaching Stretches

Reaching Above the Head
Students stand with their feet a few centimetres apart, arms extended above the head, fingers spread. Feet remain on the floor. Ask them to imagine that they are trying to reach up to the ceiling, out through the ceiling and up to the sky. With the feet apart, arms raised and fingers spread, they stretch up, up as far as they can. Hold. Let go and relax. Now ask them to see if they can stretch a little further. Repeat once more.

Stretching Sideways
Feet will be positioned as before, with arms and fingers extended. Ask students to imagine that they are trying to reach out to the walls and beyond. Start the stretch. With feet apart, arms out, fingers spread, they stretch out, out, out, to the walls as far as they can go. Hold. Let it go and relax. Repeat twice more and encourage students to reach out a little further with each stretch.

Stretching Out in Front
With feet a few centimetres apart, students extend fingers, hands and arms out to the front, at shoulder height. Start the stretch by asking the students to reach far, far into the distance. Hold the stretch. Now let it go. Repeat twice. Encourage them to reach out a little further with each stretch.

Reaching Down

With feet a few centimetres apart, tummy and bottom held in, fingers, arms and hands stretching down, students bend gently from the waist, reaching down through the floor, right down into the ground. Ask them to stretch down, down, down. Hold the stretch. Now let it go. Repeat twice. Encourage them to reach down a little further with each stretch.

Climbing Stretch

With each exercise, the students are to imagine that they are climbing up and out of their bodies.

1 Students stand with legs about 10 cm apart, arms loosely by their sides. Ensure that they are relaxed in this position. They extend arms out in front at shoulder height with fingers spread. Ask them to push the right arm up and out from the shoulder in a lifting, rolling movement as if they are climbing out of quicksand; then do this with the left arm. Alternate each arm five times.

2 With feet as above, and arms, hands and fingers extended to the sides at shoulder height, students push up and out in a rolling action to the right side, then to the left. Encourage them to lean into the action and to imagine they are climbing out to each side. Repeat five times.

3 Standing on their toes, legs 10 cm apart, arms, hands and fingers extended above their heads, students reach up and roll out of their shoulders. Ask them to imagine that they are climbing up, up and out of their bodies. First to the right then to the left. Repeat five times.

4 Students sit on the floor with legs outstretched in front. Arms, hands and fingers are extended at shoulder height in front of them. They roll shoulders, waist and hips in a climbing motion reaching out to the front, then to the right, then to the left. Repeat five times.

It is important to follow all segments of stretching with a loosening-up exercise. For example, ask students to give their bodies a gentle shake, or gently shake the individual parts of the body — the head, shoulders, arms, legs, hands, feet. Or ask them to do a body swing: with feet 30 cm apart students hold their arms out a few centimetres. They then gently swing their arms around the body.

Brick Wall Stretch

The following exercises are done with the feet placed firmly on the floor about 10 cm apart. The students imagine that they are trying to push over a big brick wall, so that each stretch needs to be a very strong one.

Front Stretch

With arms at shoulder height, hands bent up from the wrist, fingers straight and together, students imagine that there is a big red-brick wall in front of them. Get them to see the wall in their mind. Stretching out their arms, they are to push the wall, push, push, push the wall, then relax, arms dropping to the side. Repeat five times, relaxing after each stretch.

Upwards Stretch

With arms and hands above their heads, the students push against the brick wall above their heads. They try to push the wall away. Stretch up, up, up and push the wall away. Relax, with arms dropping loosely. Repeat five times, relaxing after each stretch.

Side Stretch

The big red brick wall is now at the side and the students turn from the waist to push against it. With both arms out at shoulder height, and hands bent upwards, they turn their head, shoulders and arms to the left, and stretch out, out, to push over the wall. Relax, then turn to the right and repeat the action. Alternate left and right, repeating each stretch five times, relaxing between each stretch. Finish with a gentle stretch.

Elastic Stretch

Students lie on their backs with feet about 5 cm apart, arms extended above the head in a relaxed position. Ask them to imagine they have a piece of elastic tied to their toes and to their fingers and they are going to S-T-R-E-T-C-H the elastic as far as they can and hold it, S-T-R-E-T-C-H 1 . . . 2 . . . 3 . . . 4 . . . 5. Now let the stretch go and RELAX. Repeat, gradually increasing the count to ten.

The same exercise can be repeated lying on tummies, resting foreheads flat on the floor. When the routine is completed, the students lie in their space, relaxing.

Creeping Stretch

This is a gentle stretching exercise. Students stand with feet 10 cm apart, hands on knees or thighs. Ask them to creep their hands slowly up their bodies, up, up, above their heads to the ceiling. H-O-L-D and then let arms relax and F-L-O-P forward, gently swinging arms backwards and forwards to loosen up. Repeat five times.

Cross Stretch

Students lie on their backs, feet a few centimetres apart, arms extended out from shoulders. Ask students to stretch down through their bodies to their toes and out across their bodies to their fingertips; H-O-L-D and S-T-R-E-T-C-H to a count of five and then R-E-L-A-X. Repeat five times.

The same exercise can be repeated lying on tummies with forehead resting on the floor. When the exercise is completed, ask the students to lie in their own space, turn head to side and R-E-L-A-X.

Cat Stretch

Students kneel and then sit back on heels, hands resting on thighs. Slowly push hands down thighs and along the floor, S-T-R-E-T-C-H as far as possible. Forehead comes down to rest on the floor. Hold a few seconds, then gradually push back and return to sitting position. Repeat five times.

Body Stretch

This exercise can be done sitting, lying or standing. However, when it is done lying, a greater stretch is usually achieved and people are more comfortable.

Ask the students to think of and concentrate on the muscles in their faces and to S-T-R-E-T-C-H them in any way they like. The stretching action should result in them pulling faces or having a forced smile. Gradually move down through the body, neck, shoulders, arms, hands, fingers, chest, tummy, bottom, thighs, lower legs, feet and toes. Repeat the instructions, to think of and concentrate on those muscles, and S-T-R-E-T-C-H them in any way they like. End the routine with a full body stretch, S-T-R-E-T-C-H-I-N-G all the muscles in their bodies. Finish by asking the students to R-E-L-A-X in their own space.

Note on Sitting

When doing exercises while seated it is important that children sit correctly. To do this, feet should be flat on the floor and a few centimetres apart. If the chair is too high a cushion or book can be put under the feet. (Alternatively, move forward on the chair, although this is not the best option as it is difficult to sit up straight without a back support.) Bottom is flat on the chair and the back is resting against the back of the chair. Head is straight, shoulders and back are straight but not tight or tense. Hands gently rest on the thighs. Always check that the body is in alignment and straight and that no part is held tightly.

Loosening-up Routines

These exercises complement the stretching exercises. They can be done before the stretching or instead as a separate routine. They can be done standing or sitting (see Note on Sitting above).

Head

Gently shake side to side, up and down. G-E-N-T-L-Y drop the head on to the chest, and then on to the shoulders. Repeat three or four times.

Neck

S-L-O-W-L-Y turn the head to the right as far as possible, then to the left. Now move the head around in a clockwise direction, and then anti-clockwise.

Shoulders

S-L-O-W-L-Y lift the shoulders up to the ears and G-E-N-T-L-Y let them drop down. Shake the shoulders, then lift the left up and down, the right up and down, both up and down. G-E-N-T-L-Y push each shoulder forwards, now backwards, now shake them. Roll shoulders forwards, then backwards, now G-E-N-T-L-Y shake.

Arms, Hands, Fingers

S-T-R-E-T-C-H arms forward from the shoulders, palms upwards. Bend arms at the elbow to touch the shoulders then straighten arms. Repeat five times, then gently lower arms and give them a shake. S-T-R-E-T-C-H arms forward from the shoulders, palms facing down, roll wrists one way and then back the other way, gently lower arms and shake hands. S-T-R-E-T-C-H arms forward, palms facing down, spread fingers out and open and shut them five or six times, gently shake hands.

Hold arms close to sides, elbows tucked in, G-E-N-T-L-Y push elbows out. Shoulders will also roll gently forward. Drop arms and R-E-L-A-X upper body. Swing arms around body gently.

Legs, Feet, Toes

G-E-N-T-L-Y shake legs one at a time. If sitting, G-E-N-T-L-Y kick legs forward.

Standing, feet 10 cm apart, bring right foot forward, rest on heel, toes pointing upward. G-E-N-T-L-Y move the toes up and down, then rest the foot flat. Raise toes up again, rest on heel, now spread toes out, then relax them. Next, curl toes under, then relax them. Repeat with the left foot. Finish each side with a G-E-N-T-L-E leg shake.

Stand on right leg, right hand on right knee. G-E-N-T-L-Y move the leg backwards and forwards from the knee, then circle the leg clockwise, then anticlockwise. Shake the leg. Repeat with the left leg.

If sitting, move the right leg up and down, hand on the right knee, circle leg clockwise, then anticlockwise. Repeat with left leg. Do five times.

Stand with feet about 10 cm apart, and gently swing arms around body in a circular movement, gradually making the circles bigger.

Then bring the circles slowly back smaller and smaller. Stand still and G-E-N-T-L-Y shake the upper body.

Abdomen, Tummy, Bottom

Stand with feet about 10 cm apart and G-E-N-T-L-Y push the tummy, abdomen, hips and bottom forwards and back, forwards and back. Then G-E-N-T-L-Y wiggle the bottom and shake. Repeat five times.

Body Shake

Stand with feet a little apart and G-E-N-T-L-Y shake the body up and down, shake it all over, then let the body go all floppy and R-E-L-A-X.

Again, these exercises can be done sitting or lying, and they can be selected as part of a routine or done as individual exercises. They are especially helpful for children when they need to calm down after experiencing a heightened emotional state, for example anger, excitement, frustration or anxiety.

Breathing Exercises

Relax Breathing

Students sit in their own space with their eyes closed. Legs are straight out in front of the body with the hands on thighs. The students breathe in and out slowly through their noses. Tell them: 'We are now going to inhale through our noses while I count to four. Hold your breath for four seconds, then breathe out saying the word RELAX silently finishing by the letter "X"'. Repeat five times, each time lengthening the word RELAX. Ask students to let their breathing return to normal, open their eyes and gently move their head and shoulders.

Slow Breathing

1 Count slowly in your head 1 — AND — 2 — AND — 3 — AND — etc. (The count for this exercise is slow. '1 — AND' takes about 5 seconds.) Breathe in (inhale) on 1, and breathe out (exhale) on AND. Breathe in 2, — breathe out AND. Continue the count up to 10, and then let breathing return to normal.

2 This exercise has no count. Instead it uses a simple action of the tongue to slow down the rate of breathing. Inhale, and the tongue slowly moves to the roof of the mouth. Exhale, and the tongue slowly returns to its normal resting position. Continue for ten breaths and then let the breathing go back to its normal rate.

3 Students lie in their own space in a relaxed position checking their bodies for tight spots. Ask them to inhale slowly to a count of 3, hold for 3 and exhale to a count of 3. Rest for 3, then repeat, increasing the

count by one each time. Eventually breathing should go up to a count of 10, but this very much depends on the nature of your group, so observe and be guided by them.

Deep Breathing

Students lie, relaxed, in their own space, checking that there are no tight spots. They inhale, breathe in slowly and deeply, and send the breath deep down into their toes. Then they exhale slowly, sending the breath up from their toes, right through their bodies and out. Repeat five times.

Cleansing Breathing

This breathing is used to get stale air out of our lungs and clean them out. It is a very good breathing exercise to use when we get up in the morning. It is also good to use if you are tired or have been working for a long period.

1 **Gentle**: Students stand in their own space, with legs about 10 cm apart, hands at sides. They bend from the waist and take arms to the floor and, as they do, slowly breathe out all the stale air. When their arms reach the floor and their lungs are empty, they cross over arms and come up inhaling, bringing arms up in a circle until above the head. Count to 7. As arms come down to sides, students push their breath out slowly through their mouths until their arms touch their sides. Count to 4. Wait 1-2 seconds. Repeat five times.

2 **Hard**: Students stand, feet 10 cm apart, hands on thighs. Inhale through the nose and slowly lift arms above the head. Hold the breath for 3-4 seconds, now lower arms and bring the upper body forward quickly, but gently, exhaling at the same time. This breathing out will create a 'Ha-a' sound. Rest. Then, gently uncurl the body to the initial upright position. Repeat 3-4 times.

3 **Sigh**: Students stand with feet 10 cm apart, hands loosely by their sides. Slowly inhale through the nose and lift the shoulders, hold the breath and keep the shoulders raised for a few seconds, and then exhale through the mouth with a **long sigh, relaxing the shoulders**. Repeat five times.

Energy Breathing

This breathing helps us to recharge our bodies and minds after exercise or long periods of work.

The children lie in their own space, relaxing, checking for tight spots. They concentrate on their breathing for 30 seconds. Ask them to imagine now that their breath is golden energy, like a bright golden light. This will recharge their bodies. They slowly breathe in and take the golden energy down through their bodies. They send it into each part of the body: arms, fingers, chest, legs, feet, toes.

They flood their bodies with the golden energy. Then they breathe out slowly and take the stale air out, pushing it out of their bodies, out through the top of their heads. Repeat this exercise five times, talking the children through it each time.

Guided Imagery Exercises

These can be used as part of a short routine, which could include stretching, muscle and breathing work. They can be done either sitting or lying. Refer to Session Seven, page 57, Quiet Time exercise for details of setting the scene and the finishing routine, which ends each exercise.

Setting the Scene

Have Quiet Time music playing softly. Ask the children to take themselves to their special place. Remember to speak slowly, add your own pauses and repeat key words or sentences.

Doing Something Well

Today in our special place we are going to practise doing something we **really want to do well**. Now, think about the thing you want to do well and in your mind make a statement about it like 'I will read really well'. Now, leave what you are lying on and start practising what you are doing really well. See yourself — you are doing a fantastic job, hear yourself, feel yourself doing it and tell yourself, 'I can do this... really well'. Keep on practising and talking to yourself, telling yourself how well you can do that special thing. Now, finish what you are doing, S-L-O-W-L-Y go back and lie on your special something and R-E-L-A-X in your special place, **feeling calm and peaceful and confident. Remember**, you can do things really well; just **relax, talk** to yourself and **practise** in your mind.

Being Peaceful

Today in your special place, you are going to concentrate on being peaceful. You are going to make your mind and body still and quiet and peaceful, a beautiful, strong, calm peacefulness will become part of you, something you can feel whenever you want.

Now let all your muscles relax and slow your breathing down. Feel the breath coming in, filling up your lungs and flowing through your body. As you breathe in, you feel your body warm and full of peace, your muscles are floppy, your mind is still, your breath is slow and **peace fills you up** and spreads down through your body. **You feel so great, calm and peaceful, happy and relaxed.**

Now I want you to stay with that feeling, **relax**, listen to the music and just feel **calm and peaceful, and remember** — you can feel this way any time you choose; just use your breathing and your wonderful brain to help you. Now **relax and feel calm and peaceful**.

Feeling Free

Today in your special place you are going to practise feeling free; free from anything that has been worrying you or making you sad, angry, frightened or hurt. Now think about what you want to be **free** from, say it to yourself: '**I will be free from . . .**' As you inhale, feel your breath coming in. You are going to feel free. Free from your worry, your anger, hurt, fear, whatever you want. As you exhale, feel your problem leaving you, see it floating up and away, away. Say to yourself, '**I am free**' then, 'I am free from . . .' Breathe in slowly and stay with the feeling, free, peaceful, happy, still and quiet.

Remember, you can be free any time you want. You can choose to tell yourself: '**I am free**' and be really **free**. Rest now. Listen to the music. Feel wonderful.

Rested and Energized

Today in your special place you are going to get rid of all your tiredness and become full of energy. Golden energy will fill your body and it will feel **rested, calm and peaceful**. It has been a hot/cold, busy/long, day, and your whole body has been active doing all the things you have had to do, running, playing, working, eating, thinking.

Now it's time to rest, to let all the action and busy work go. So send out a big breath, let it out of your body, let all the muscles go floppy, and relax and slow your breathing down, feeling the breath come in and fill up your body. Slowly the tiredness begins to melt **away, away out of your body**, each part is **relaxed and resting**. Feel your body resting; make a picture in your mind of yourself **resting, calm and peaceful**. Now as you breathe in you bring in **golden energy**. It fills your body, making it glow. Your body is rested and now it is filling up with **golden energy**. Feel it and see the beautiful **golden energy** flowing into your body with each breath.

Now remember you can rest your body and fill it up with energy. Just use your brain and your golden breath and be still and quiet. Now listen to the music and think about your **wonderful rested and energized body. Don't forget to feel it and to see yourself rested and calm and peaceful.**

Boss of Your Feelings

Today in your special place you are going to be boss of your feelings. I want you to think about a feeling you get that sometimes makes you feel uncomfortable. Now think about when you feel this way. Think about who is there and what is happening but, most importantly, see it all in your mind. What part of your body has the feeling? Your head?

Your tummy? Your chest? Where is that feeling in your body? You need to know because you are going to make that feeling small. You are going to be boss of that feeling, because when your feelings make you feel uncomfortable they are getting too big and they are starting to be the boss of you. You need to tell those feelings you are **the boss ... you can make your body strong and calm**. Say that slowly to yourself now: 'I can be boss of my ...' Say it twice more. Let your muscles be floppy and relaxed and feel yourself being **boss of that feeling by making it smaller and smaller** until it is just the right size and you are boss.

Rest now. Listen to the music and feel **calm, powerful and strong and boss of your feeling and peaceful.**

Part Four

HELPING YOUR CHILD TO RELAX

Ideas for Parents

In this section I have attempted to provide you with some additional
ideas to help your child. If you feel that the program presented in Part
Two of the book would not fit in with your lifestyle, or that your child
or yourself are not quite ready for that approach, don't give up; there
are simple things you can do to help your child become a more relaxed
person.

First and foremost, you need to be a **role model of the behaviour**
you wish your child to adopt. If you take a **more relaxed approach
to life**, in time your child will too. Try stepping back from situations.
Here is a simple plan to help you:

- **Stop** — slow your breathing down and let go of your tight 'ouch' spots
  — they are the muscles you hold tight when you become anxious,
  angry, worried or upset.
- **Think** — what is really happening in this situation? Check your
  information and don't make assumptions. You might be wrong about
  things. The situation might not be as you see it.
- **Act** — after you have done the above, choose your action, **don't just
  respond**; act in an informed, thoughtful way.

Look at the demands being placed on your child: by yourself, other
people and herself or himself. If, on reflection, you feel there are too
many demands, then talk to your child and the people involved, and
make some suggestions or changes to lessen the demands. For example,
think about the number of after-school activities your child is involved
in, if you feel there are too many look at ways of rationalizing them.
Your child does not have to do something every day. Help your child to
manage his or her time by providing guidelines, structure and time
limits, but make sure there is still time for leisure or just 'mucking
around'. Try to remember that children **do not need to be busy all
the time**. Practise this philosophy yourself and see that your child
understands and practises it also.

Give your child the opportunity to increase coping skills. Help your
child to use positive self-talk, to develop responsibility and the ability
to make decisions. In practical terms, ensure that your child has a

balanced diet and sleeps regular, adequate hours. These things will assist your child to develop a more positive approach to his or her own well- being.

Develop some simple Quiet Time routines, for example, sitting together reading, giving your child a massage, listening to quiet music or a guided imagery exercise together or sharing a meditation exercise such as those suggested in *Starbright* and *Sweet Dreams Little Ones* (see References and Further Reading).

Try some short routine activities which you can select from Part Three.

However, before you do this, I would like to encourage you to teach and share with your child the basic skill of being able to be in **one's own space** and understanding **one's own body, breathing and muscles** and how to use **one's own imagination**. This can be done in a less formal way than suggested in the text, but can still be of great benefit to your child, as it will help the child to develop the skill of learning to use **relaxation** to help respond to life's demands.

Simple Activities for Home

- Loosening up.
- Stretching.
- Making tight and floppy shapes.
- Tighten and relax the whole body.
- Put on some quiet music, sit in a comfortable position and just relax and listen.
- Sit cross-legged on the floor facing each other with knees touching. With your hands on your child's knees, both of you close your eyes and slow your breathing down to breathe in time to the music. Keep that position for about 4-5 minutes. Gently stand and stretch and give each other a hug. A variation is to sit behind your child and place your hands on his or her shoulders.
- Your child lies in his or her own space, gently stroke or massage the back while listening to the music. Always end with a stretch and a hug.

Massage

Another activity, which is a wonderful way of helping children to be more relaxed and to become more aware of their bodies, in particular their tension 'ouch' spots, is **massage**. It has been acknowledged by many authorities that massage can bring comfort, calmness, reassurance and relief from tension. Also, since massage involves gentle physical contact, it can be a means of strengthening your relationship with your child and may revive some of that wonderful closeness you had when he or she was a baby. Then, as you went about their daily care, your interaction involved much more stroking, patting and touching.

Before beginning any massage activity, make sure you are in a warm, quiet place and that your hands are clean and warm. Your fingernails need to be short, and do not wear jewellery. Avoid talking, and concentrate on your movements, keeping your hands relaxed and sensitive.

Check that your child is comfortable in his or her physical, seeing, hearing and mind space. It is useful to play some gentle, flowing music softly in the background. Ask him or her to close the eyes as you do the massage. All the movements in the exercises can be repeated as many times as you wish, but remember to have a firm but gentle touch.

Scalp Massage

Your child sits in a comfortable position either on the floor or with back support on a chair. You kneel or sit behind, with your hands placed gently on top of the child's head. Start with a firm, stroking motion and move from the top of the head, down the back and then around to the side and to the front. Now take your hands to the centre of the head and gently massage the scalp as if you are shampooing the hair. Move your fingertips all around, down the side of the scalp, the front and the back. Now repeat the stroking movement, down the back, the side and the front. Return to the side and finally to the back, and slowly bring your hands down and rest them on your child's shoulders. Just be still and quiet for a few seconds.

Face and Forehead

Adopt a comfortable position for yourself and your child and have your child gently close his or her eyes. Now, gently using your fingertips in a circular movement, start at the centre of the forehead and move outwards and around the outline of your child's face, ending at the chin. Move back up the face to the forehead.

Change the movement by gently pressing your fingertips into the surface, move around the outline of the face again and return to the forehead. Cupping your hands, stroke the forehead from the eyebrows upwards to the hairline, moving across the forehead and back again. Now take the middle three fingers down to the eyelids. Gently press and pat the area around the eyes, temples, nose, cheeks, mouth and chin.

Move back up the face again, ending at the forehead. Gently stroke the whole face, using circular and downward movements. End the massage by resting your hands on your child's head or shoulders for a few seconds.

Neck

Adopt a comfortable position for you and your child. To start, ask your child to gently move the neck by slowly turning the head from side to side, chin up and down gently, shoulders up and down. Now gently stroke your child's head. Now, with your fingertips, start at the base of the head, gently pressing up and down, and around the base of the neck. Continue by moving around to the front of the neck, but make sure that the finger pressure is only slight on this area. Return to the back, use a circular movement, gradually moving down and around the back neck area.

Move to the front of the neck and use a stroking movement, gently up and down, covering the whole area. Now move to the back of the neck and continue this stroking movement out over the shoulders. End the massage by gently resting your hands on the child's shoulders.

Shoulders

Position your child lying face downwards. Place a small flat cushion or pillow under the abdomen and ankles (this is more comfortable and lessens the possibility of arching and tensing the back). Place both hands at the base of the child's spine with your fingers pointing upwards and your hands flat. Working alongside the spine (not on it) move your hands up, gently grasping the skin in a creeping type of movement.

Work right up the back and over the shoulders. Moulding your hand to the contours of the back, move back down the back to the base.

Hand massage

Adopt a comfortable sitting position for yourself and your child. Ask your child to shake the hands slowly and then to rest them on the thighs. Slowly and gently take one hand, holding the palm face up. Now gently but firmly, using both your thumbs, massage the palm of your child's hand by pressing into it and moving around the whole area.

Move up to the little finger, pressing from the base to the tip and back down again. Gently stroke up from the back and then the side of the finger. Do each finger the same way. Rub the hand all over, both the front and the back. Repeat the same series of movements with the other hand. Finish the massage by gently holding your child's hands in yours for a few seconds, then let the hands return to your child's thighs.

Road Massage

This is a fun activity that can be done in pairs or as a family group. I always use it in my adult stress management and relaxation groups as it adds a lighthearted touch to a session.

Sit in a line on the floor with backs exposed. Tell the participants that you are going to pretend that their backs are pieces of land which are going to be made into roads and that your hands are going to do the work. (If you are doing it in a group, one person can demonstrate out the front on the back of a volunteer while giving the following instructions.) Remember to make the movements FIRM BUT GENTLE.

- First we are going to dig up the road using our thumbs, DIG, DIG, DIG.
- Then we put the tar on the road, PAT, PAT, PAT.
- Next we will roll the tar on the road, ROLL, ROLL, ROLL.
- Now we will put the line down the middle, FINGER GENTLY MOVES ALONG SPINE.
- Now we will plant the trees along the side of the road, DIG AND PAT, DIG AND PAT, DIG AND PAT.
- Finally, along come the cars, SWISH, SWISH, SWISH (use opposing hand movements).

My thanks to Judith Gray, educator at the Centre for Social Health at Fairfield Hospital in Melbourne, for allowing me to include this exercise in this text.

Part Five

HOLDING A PARENT INFORMATION WORKSHOP

It is of great importance to try to engage the parents of the children with whom you are working. In my experience, the parents who are informed and can actively support your work will assist their children and, in turn, these children will gain more from the program.

The parent night needs to be held before the program begins or, at the latest, in the first week. You need to plan for a two-hour workshop. A suggested format you might like to follow and the overheads you will need are included in this part of the book. I also strongly encourage you to take the parents through some practical exercises. In my experience, the parents respond very positively to this activity and they gain an additional insight into how you will be working with the children.

At the end of this section, there are some useful handout notes to give to parents at the end of a children's program.

SUGGESTED FORMAT

Purpose of the Information Night
- To provide parents with information about the program's concepts and skills taught and how the program will be presented.
- To encourage a cooperative relationship between parents and teachers.

Outline for the Evening
- Introduce the course leader.
- Present the aims of the program, which are to give the children the opportunity to:
—increase their coping skills so they can respond to the demands of their lives;
—build an awareness and understanding of their wonderful bodies and how they work;
—learn how to make their bodies **calm** and **peaceful**. (Use Overhead 15.)

Theory Behind the Program

The distress we feel in many life situations is often the result of the interaction between an individual's coping skills and the demands of the environment (Overhead 16). Therefore, we need to encourage children to increase their repertoire of coping skills so that they can respond constructively to such demands (Overhead 17). Give the example of the child who has to read at the school assembly. (See the introduction to this book.)

Concepts and Skills Taught

Introduce the definition of *relaxation* used in the program. (Use Overhead 1).

- Discuss concept of program and skills taught. (Use Overhead 14.)
- How the sessions are structured. (Use Overheads 18 and 19.)
- Provide some practical exercises.

Before beginning these activities, introduce the idea that relaxation is a process and that lying down listening to a quiet music tape is really the last phase. Talk about the importance of the preparation stage, then the relaxation routine. (Use Overhead 20.)

Activities

1 Select a stretching and cleansing breathing exercise from Part Three.

2 Demonstrate how to lie in your own space. Let participants try the positions and have them adopt one which is comfortable for them. Move on to the relaxation routine.

3 Select a muscle-relaxing exercise, then a breathing exercise and finally a guided imagery exercise. I usually use the one in Session Seven on page 57 or, if I have more time, a longer one. If you are not fully confident, use one of the commercial tapes suggested on page 101.

Benefits of Relaxation Routine

1 Spend a few minutes discussing the participants' responses to the practical activities.

2 Briefly discuss the benefits of a relaxation routine. (Use Overhead 21.)

How to Use the Workbook

Have copies of the Workbook available for parents to look at, and discuss with them ways they might work through the book with their child. This is very important if you have decided to let parents introduce the Workbook to their child.

Notes for Parents

Helping Your Child to Relax

Parents often ask what **they** can do to continue the work when the ten sessions of relaxation classes have finished.

The most important thing is to have faith in your ability to continue the child's skill development. The skills the child has learnt and practised in the group are basic, and all the students have acquired some degree of competence in using them. All she or he needs now is your interest, support, guidance and help to use these skills in everyday life.

What You Can Do

- Be aware of the theory behind the program: how our thoughts and feelings contribute to our behaviour. Relaxation skills are positive behaviour. They are a constructive reaction that will assist us when we respond to a happening in our daily life. This behaviour helps us to make our whole body calm and peaceful.
- Remind your child often that she or he has a wonderful body and should treat it **gently**. Also remind your child that she or he can get the body to work in **harmony**, that is, the inside and outside parts working together.
- Monitor your own body and find out where you hold your tension. These will be your **ouch** spots. Be observant of your child. It is most likely that she or he will have similar 'ouch' spots. Observe and encourage your child and, if need be, help her or him to let go. Gently stroking or just touching will help your child to let go those tight 'ouch' spots.
- Encourage your child to practise making her or his body tight and then letting it become loose and floppy. The child can become:
  — a tall, straight, light post;
  — a wobbly, wobbly jelly fish;
  — a tight, tight spring;
  — a loose, loose overcoat.
  During the ten weeks we have learnt how to stretch our bodies and how to loosen up our head, neck, shoulders, arms, hands, fingers, legs, feet, etc. Encourage your child to practise these exercises.
- Remind and help your child to practise the various breathing exercises she or he has learnt.

Slow Breathing. This can be done to a count of ten: 1 ... 2 ... 3 ... 4 inhale; 6 ... 7 ... 8 ... 9 ... 10 exhale. Encourage your child to concentrate quietly and slow the breathing.

Relax breathing is another deep breathing exercise. Slowly inhale and exhale, saying the word RELAX.

Cleansing breathing is filling our lungs and then pushing out all the stale air.

Energy breathing recharges our internal organs. When we do energy breathing we inhale a deep breath, bringing in golden energy and we send it down through our body, to the soles of our feet, slowly exhaling.

Slow and relax breathing are used to calm ourselves, when we are anxious, frightened, overtired, out of breath, or to help us to get to sleep.

Cleansing breathing is best done in the mornings. It cleans out our lungs and revitalizes us.

Energy breathing helps to recharge us if we are tired. It can be used as a motivation to get ourselves ready for work or to do a task we don't like.

- Encourage your child to use her or his brain to create positive pictures in the mind. These pictures can assist us in many, many situations. We call these pictures *images*. We can create an image of our own special place, where we can create images of ourselves being wonderful and special people. We can also create positive images of ourselves to assist us when we are anxious, angry or need to feel special.

- Finally, **remind** your child **often** that she or he:
  — has a wonderful body that can work in **harmony**;
  — can make herself or himself **calm** and **peaceful**;
  — should treat the body **gently**;
  — is a **special person**;
  — should give herself or himself a hug often.
  AND YOU GIVE THE CHILD ONE TOO.

MUSIC

Music should be quiet and gentle and have little variation in tempo. Here are some suggestions for tapes and CDs and where you can obtain them.

- *Tranquillity*, Sun Productions, 1989.
- *Fairy Ring*, Mike Rowland, New World Productions, 1982.
- *Silver Wings*, Mike Rowland, New World Productions, 1985.
- *Butterfly*, Jeff Clarkson, Gateway Productions, 1986.
- *Gentle Sounds*, Carey Landry, Side 1, Track 2, 'Peace is Flowing Like a River', Epoch Universal Publications, 1987.

Available from:
St Paul Book and Media Centre, 7 Denmark Hill Road, East Hawthorn Vic. 3122. Ph: (03) 882 3424.
Chrysalis Bookshop, 245A Glenferrie Road, Malvern Vic. 3144.
Ph: (03) 509 2310.

- *James Galway's Greatest Hits* Vol. 1 & 2; especially 'Annie's song' and 'Song of the seashore'.
Available from major music stores.

Tapes with Spoken Imagery Dialogue

- *Deep Relaxation/Dolphin Cycle*, Sally Kirk, Golden Cassettes, 1986.
- *Your Special Place*, Sally Kirk, Golden Cassettes, 1984.
- *Just Imagine*, Anthea Courtenay, Golden Cassettes, 1983.

Available from Golden Cassettes, C/o the Relaxation Centre of Queensland, Cnr Brookes and Wickham Streets, Fortitude Valley Qld 4006. Ph: (07) 252 4157.

- *Let's Imagine*, Verity James, Magic Music.
- *Let's Imagine — The Crystal Castle*, Allan Symonds, Magic Music.

Available from Magic Music, PO Box 62, North Perth WA 6006.
Ph: (09) 271 4357.

Some Other Stockists for Relaxation and Meditation Music and Books

Victoria
Esoteric Bookshop, Glen Arcade, 675 Glenferrie Road, Hawthorn Vic. 3122. Ph: (03) 818 1998.
Open Leaves Bookshop, 71 Cardigan Street, Carlton Vic. 3053. Ph: (03) 347 2355.
Theosophical Society Bookshop, 2nd Floor, 128 Russell Street, Melbourne Vic. 3000. Ph: (03) 650 3955.

New South Wales
Adyar Bookshop, 230 Clarence Street, Sydney NSW 2000. Ph: (02) 267 8509.
New Awareness Centre and Bookshop, 302 Pacific Highway, Lindfield NSW 2070. Ph: (02) 416 3938.
Sydney Esoteric Bookshop, 408 Elizabeth Street, Surry Hills NSW 2010. Ph: (02) 212 2225.

Northern Territory
Agni Bookshop, Wulagi Shopping Centre, Wulagi, Darwin NT 0812. Ph: (089) 45 2774.
Parap Secondhand Bookshop, Parap Shopping Village, Parap, Darwin NT 0820. Ph: (089) 81 3922.

South Australia
Adelaide Theosophical Bookshop, 334 King William Street, Adelaide SA 5000. Ph: (08) 212 5356.
COPE Bookshop, 116 Hutt Street, Adelaide SA 5000. Ph: (08) 223 3433.
Quantum Bookshop, 113 Melbourne Street, North Adelaide SA 5006. Ph: (08) 267 1579.

Western Australia
New Age Media, 3 Pakenham Street, Fremantle WA 6160. Ph: (09) 430 4305.
Perth Theosophical Society Bookshop, 21 Glendower Street, Perth WA 6000. Ph: (09) 328 8104.

Queensland
Brisbane Theosophical Bookstore, 355 Wickham Terrace, Brisbane Qld 4000. Ph: (07) 839 1453.
New World Productions, PO 244, Red Hill, Brisbane, Qld 4059. Ph: (07) 367 0788.
Vicki Bennett Training, PO 1940, Brisbane Qld 4001. Ph: (07) 831 1082.

Tasmania
Akashic Bookshop, 26F Cat and Fiddle Arcade, 101 Collins Street, Hobart Tas. 7000. Ph: (002) 23 8524

FURTHER READING

Buxbaum S. K. and Gelman R. G. (1984), *Body Noises*. Hamish Hamilton, London.

Cook, R. (1988), *Relaxation for Children*. SBRP Health Handbook. Second Back Row Press, Katoomba.

Kipper, I. (1980), *My Magic Garden: A Meditation Guide for Children*. Pathways Press, Palo Alto, California.

McKinnon, P. (1990), *Quiet Magic: A Fantasy*. David Lovell Publishing, Melbourne.

McKinnon, P. (1991), *Help Yourself and Your Child to Happiness*. David Lovell Publishing, Melbourne.

Pappas, M. G. (1982), *Sweet Dreams Little Ones*. Winston Press, Minneapolis.

Richter, B. and Jacobsen, A. (1979), *Make It So: A Child's Book on Self-direction through Affirmation*. De Vorss & Co. Marina del Rey, California.

Rozman, D. (1989), *Meditation for Children: Pathways to Happiness, Harmony, Creativity and Fun for the Family*. 2nd ed, Aslan Publishing, Boulder Creek, California.

* See page 102 for a brief selection of book stockists. Check also your local telephone directories.

Masters for
Overhead Transparencies

RELAXATION

getting our whole body to be calm and peaceful

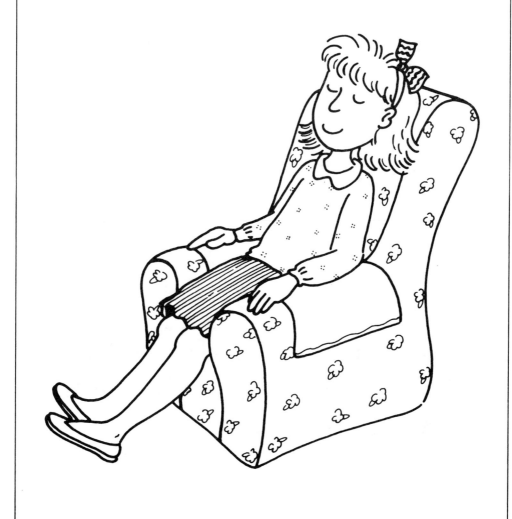

BODY HARMONY

- knowing the parts of your body and how they can work together;

- getting the inside and outside body parts working together so you can be **calm** and **peaceful.**

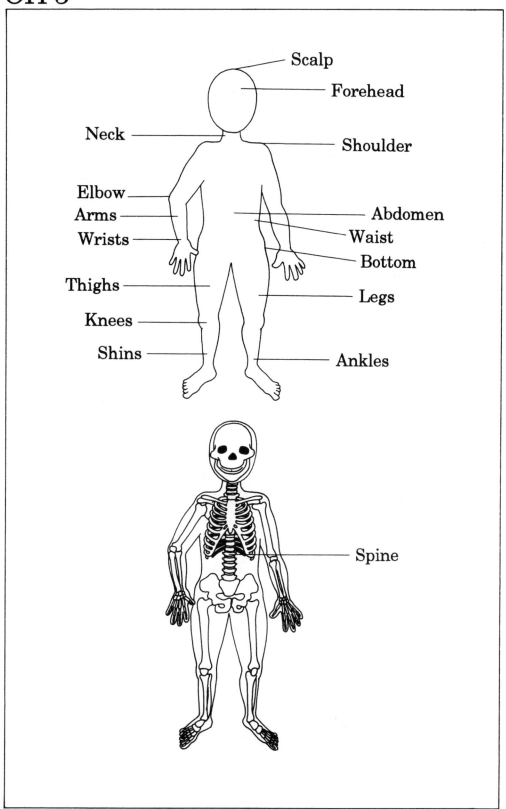

Scalp

Forehead

Neck

Shoulder

Elbow

Arms

Wrists

Abdomen

Waist

Bottom

Thighs

Legs

Knees

Shins

Ankles

Spine

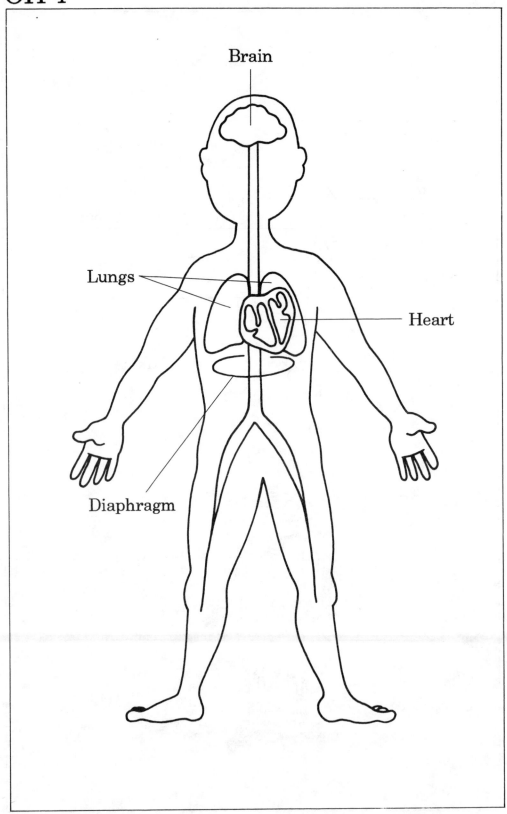

Brain

Lungs

Heart

Diaphragm

GETTING INTO MY OWN SPACE

MY OWN SPACE

- creating my *own*
  - physical
  - seeing
  - hearing
  - mind
  space;

- being able to stay in my own space so that I can be **calm** and **peaceful**.

Body Harmony

MUSCLE KNOWLEDGE

- knowing the large muscle groups and working with them;

- recognizing your **'ouch'** spots and learning how to let them go, so you can be **calm** and **peaceful**.

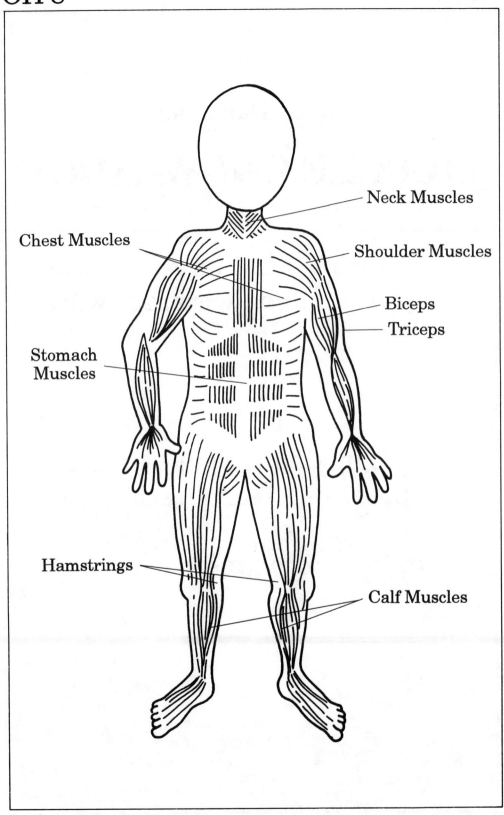

Neck Muscles

Chest Muscles

Shoulder Muscles

Biceps

Triceps

Stomach
Muscles

Hamstrings

Calf Muscles

Body Harmony

BREATHING

- knowing how we breathe and controlling our breathing;

- learning different types of breathing which will help us to be **calm** and **peaceful**.

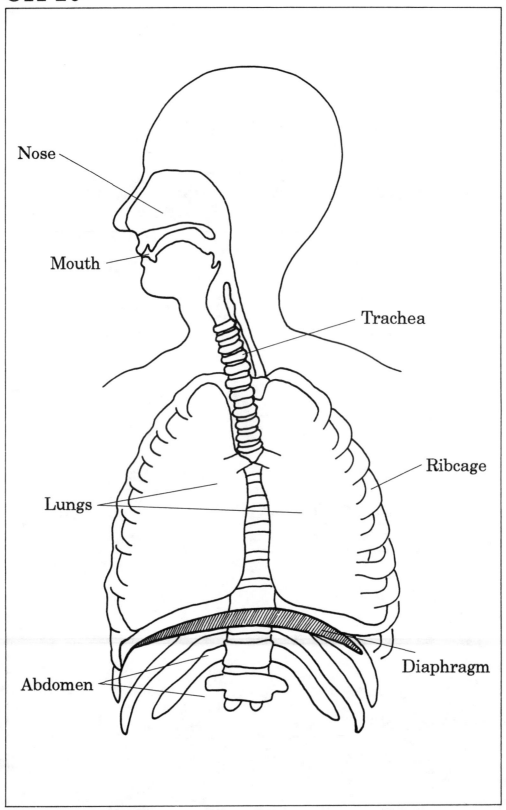

Nose

Mouth

Trachea

Ribcage

Lungs

Diaphragm

Abdomen

IMAGERY

using our brain to create pictures in our mind

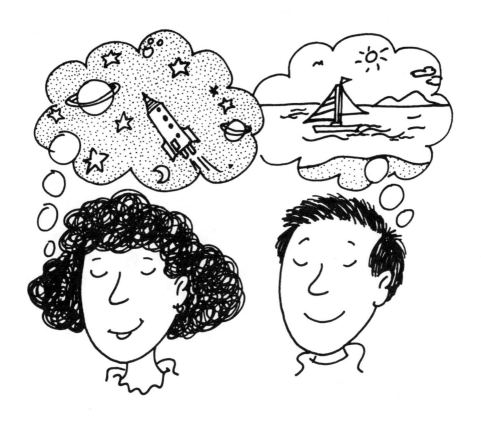

My Own Space

IMAGERY

using our brain to create pictures in our mind

These pictures can help us:

- to get our whole body to be **calm** and **peaceful**;

- to feel **great** about ourselves;

- to practise new or difficult things.

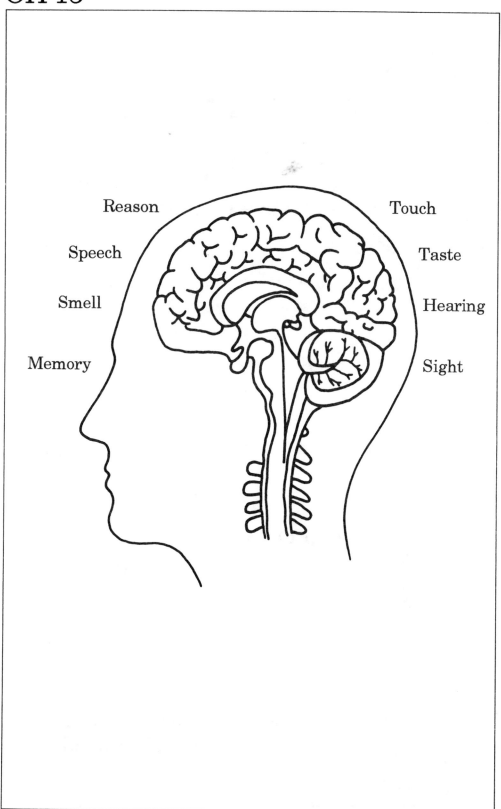

KEY CONCEPTS OF RELAXATION

**Body Harmony:
Getting the inside and outside parts
of the body working together.**

Skill Areas

- Body Knowledge   – knowing the parts of
  our body and how
  they can work together;

- Muscle Knowledge – knowing the large
  muscle groups and
  working with them;

- Breathing   – knowing how we breathe
  and controlling our
  breathing.

**Our Own Space:
Being able to be in our own space.**

Skill Areas

- Our Own Space   – creating our own physical,
  seeing, hearing, mind
  space;

- Imagery   – using our brain to create
  pictures in our mind.

THE AIMS OF THIS RELAXATION PROGRAM ARE:

- to increase students' coping skills so that they can respond positively to the demands of their lives;

- to build awareness and understanding of our wonderful bodies and how they work;

- to know how to make our whole body **calm** and **peaceful**.

DISTRESS

The gap between
the demands of
the environment and
an individual's
coping skills.

WHAT IS NEEDED

To teach children to value and enjoy a range of techniques that will help them to:

- cope with the demands of their lives;

- use stress constructively;

- develop skills that promote their own well-being.

THE SIX STAGES

1. Joining Together

This is when a 'working circle' is made; this is a way we show that we will join together and cooperate in helping each other to learn the relaxation skills and practise them.

2. Review Time

At the beginning of each session the leader and students discuss how they have practised the skills they learnt in the previous session. Time can also be spent discussing the key concepts and revising skills.

3. Instruction Time

In this segment the students are introduced to the main concepts of the program and the skills they need to acquire to be able to make their bodies and minds **calm** and **peaceful**.

4. Practical Activities

Here the students practise skills. They stretch and loosen their muscles, making their bodies tight and floppy. Deepen and slow down their breathing. Experiment with getting into their own space and use imagery to help them in all the activities.

5. Quiet Time

Quiet Time is when the students get into their **own space** and use imagery to help them to become **calm** and **peaceful** and to feel **great** about themselves.

6. Reflection

In this final stage of the session students discuss how they felt doing the activities and they are given feedback about their progress. The students also comment on how they will practise and when they will use the skills before the next session.

RELAXATION PROCESS

Preparation

- getting into own space;
- stretching;
- cleansing breathing;
- awareness of tension spots.

Relaxation Routine

- work with muscles and tension spots;
- change breathing rate;
- quiet time — using imagery and positive self-talk.

BENEFITS OF A RELAXATION ROUTINE

- promotes well-being;

- revitalizes mind and body;

- helps us to:

  - understand and read our body;

  - pick up early warning signs of our body's reactions to anxiety triggers;

  - clear our mind;

  - reduce anxiety, which can interfere with performance;

  - develop tension-reducing routines;

  - relax our body;

  - develop and use positive self-talk and imagery.

MY RELAXATION WORKBOOK

RELAXATION
getting our whole body to be calm and peaceful

This book belongs to

....

INTRODUCTION

This is your own special book about you, your body and how to **relax**.

Slowly and carefully work through each page. At the end of each section there is space for you to make your own notes. These can be things you have learnt, something you want to practise, ideas or just whatever you want to write down.

Have fun, enjoy the program and:

- get to know your body;
- always treat your body gently;
- remember you are a wonderful and special person.

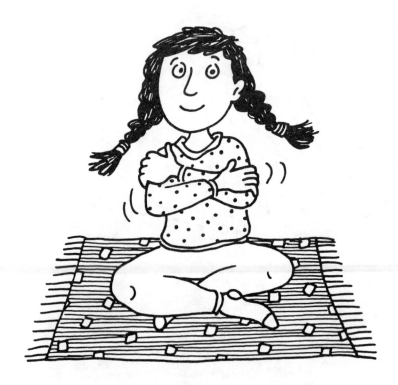

Draw a picture or paste in a photo of yourself. Then write or draw some of the things that are special about you.

GETTING INTO OUR OWN SPACE

We need to be able to get into our own:
- physical space;
- hearing space;
- seeing space;
- mind space.

When I am in *my own physical space* I am comfortable and I am not touching anyone.

When I am in *my own hearing space* I block off all sound and noise and I do not make any sounds or noises myself.

When I am in *my own seeing space* I am not looking around. I have my eyes closed.

When I am in *my own mind space* I no longer think about every-day things. My mind is blank.

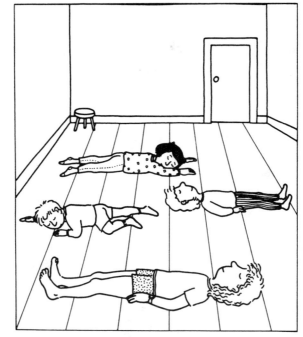

GETTING INTO MY OWN SPACE

Draw a picture of yourself in your own space:

My practice plan:

BODY HARMONY

Knowledge of your body parts: Getting the 'inside' and the 'outside' parts of your body working together.

Outside body parts we should know: **head scalp forehead cheeks neck shoulders arms wrists fingers chest abdomen waist bottom thighs shins calves ankles feet.**

We should know where these parts of our body are and what they look and feel like.

Remember:

- Know what your body looks and feels like.
- Learn the names of the different parts of your body.
- Always treat your body gently.
- You are a **wonderful** and **special** person.
- Give yourself a **hug** each day.

My own notes:

My practice plan:

Relaxation for Children © Jenny Rickard 1991, 1994. Published by ACER Ltd.

Mark and write in the names of your *outside* body parts: the ones you work with when you relax.

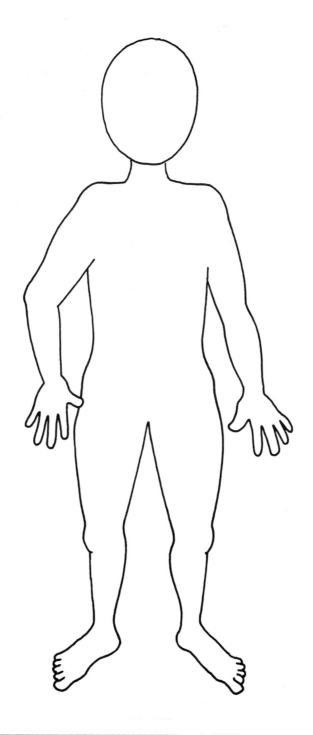

BODY HARMONY

Knowledge of your body parts: Getting the inside and the outside parts of your body working together.

Inside body parts we should know: **brain spine heart lungs diaphragm.**

We should know where these important parts are and how they work.

Remember:

- Know what your body looks and feels like.
- Learn the names of the different parts of your body.
- Always treat your body gently.
- Give yourself a hug each day.
- You are a **wonderful** and **special** person.

My own notes:

My practice plan:

Mark and write in the names of your *inside* body parts: the ones you work with when you relax.

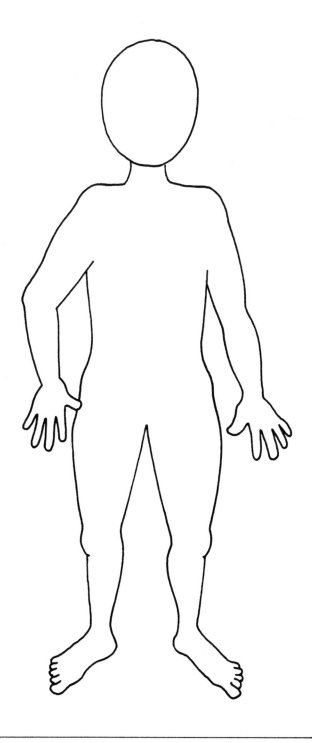

BODY HARMONY

Knowledge of your muscles:

- Knowledge of your large muscle groups and where they are and what they feel like when they are **tight** and when they are **floppy**.
- **Large Muscle Groups.** We have large muscle groups in our: **chest arms legs shoulders abdomen tummy bottom.**
  We can make these muscles **tight** or we can **relax** them and make them feel **floppy**.

Remember:

- When your muscles are **tight** they are saying **ouch**.
- Get to know where your **ouch** spots are.

My own notes:

My practice plan:

Mark in your large muscle groups: neck, chest, shoulders, triceps, biceps, stomach, hamstring, calves.

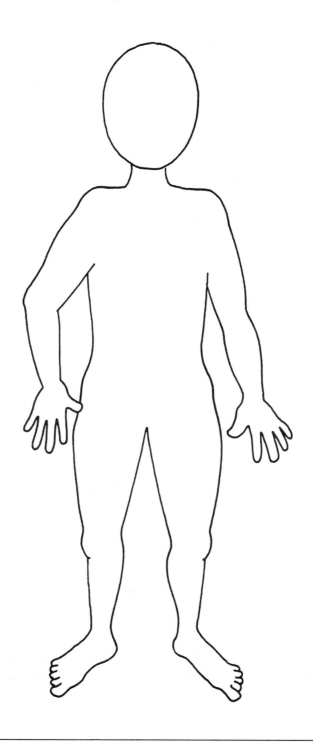

Mark in your 'ouch' spots.

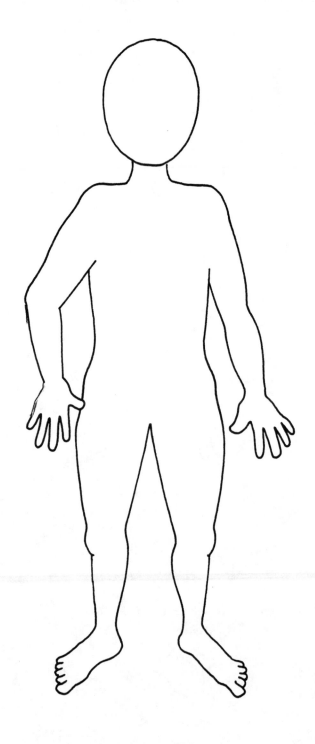

BODY HARMONY

Knowledge of how we breathe: We need to know how we breathe and how we can control our breathing to assist us when we need it.

We need to know:
- how to slow our breathing down;
- how to clean out our lungs;
- how to use our breathing to help us **relax**.

My own notes:

My practice plan:

Mark in how you breathe.

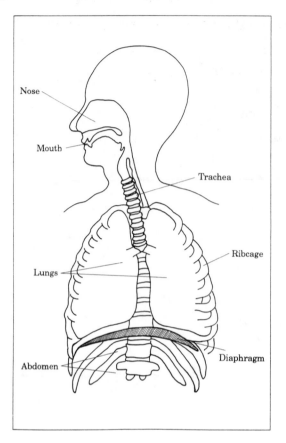

Write down or draw below what happens to your lungs when you:

Inhale

Exhale

IMAGERY
using our brain to create pictures in our mind
and
creating a mind space

Our brain is a wonderful part of our body. We can use it in many ways, some of which are:

- to help us create our own special space;
- to create a picture of ourselves doing the things we want to do;
- to help us to deal with our feelings, in particular, when we are scared, anxious, excited or unhappy.

My own notes:

My practice plan:

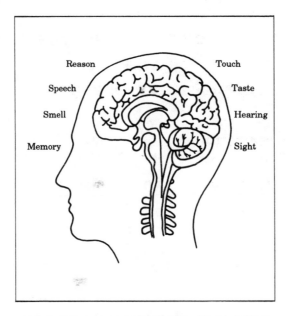

MY WONDERFUL BRAIN

IMAGERY
using our brain to create pictures in our mind.

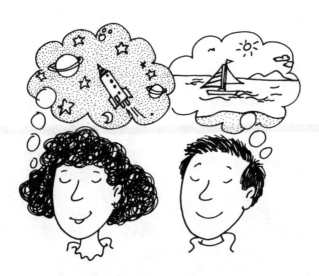

Draw or write about some images: pictures you can make with your brain.

RELAXATION

Relaxation means: Getting the whole body to be **calm** and **peaceful**.

KEY CONCEPTS OF RELAXATION

Body Harmony:
Getting the inside and outside parts
of the body working together.

Skill Areas

- Body Knowledge — knowing the parts of our body and how they can work together;
- Muscle Knowledge groups — knowing the large muscle and working with them;
- Breathing — knowing how we breathe and controlling our breathing.

Our Own Space:
Being able to be in our own space.

Skill Areas

- Our Own Space — creating our own physical, seeing, hearing, mind space;
- Imagery — using our brain to create pictures in our mind.

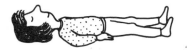

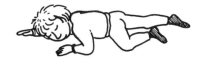

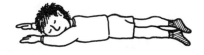

Relaxation Certificate

HAS COMPLETED A TEN WEEK COURSE IN RELAXATION

CONCEPTS I HAVE LEARNT AND SKILLS I HAVE DEVELOPED:

GETTING MY WHOLE BODY TO BE CALM AND PEACEFUL

CREATING MY OWN SPACE

MUSCLE AWARENESS

BREATHING AWARENESS

CREATING IMAGES AND LEARNING HOW TO USE IMAGERY

Teacher

Date

NOTES

NOTES